John Lane

John Lane spent 35 years in the Royal Navy where he saw operational service in Malaya, Aden and North Borneo and commanded naval establishments in Gibraltar and Oman. After leaving the Navy he served as a Senior Hospital Administrator in the Gulf War, and he has worked for the Ryder Cheshire Foundation, and for the International Red Cross in trouble spots across the world. In 1992 he was head of mission for the HALO Trust in Afghanistan. He was awarded the OBE in 1985.

A Very Peruvian Practice

Travels with La Señora

JOHN LANE

JOHN MURRAY

First published in 2003 by John Murray (Publishers)
A division of Hodder Headline

Paperback edition 2004

1 3 5 7 9 10 8 6 4 2

A CIP catalogue record for this title is available from the British
Library

ISBN 0-7195-6217 1

Typeset in Adobe Palatino by Servis Filmsetting Ltd, Manchester
Printed and bound in Great Britain by Clays Ltd, St Ives plc

John Murray (Publishers)
338 Euston Road
London
NW1 3BH

For Henrietta

Contents

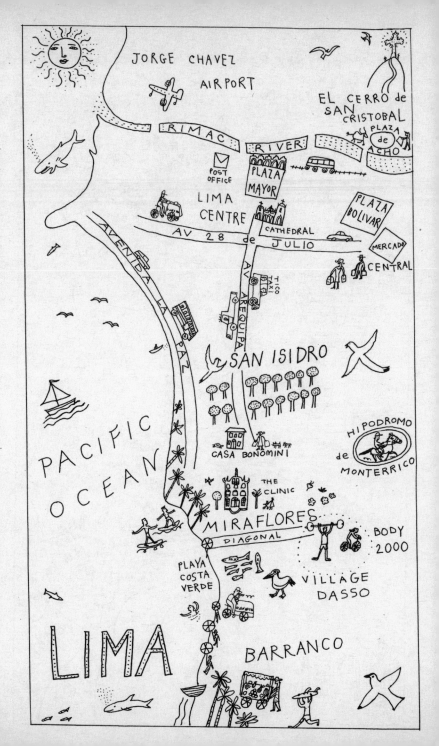

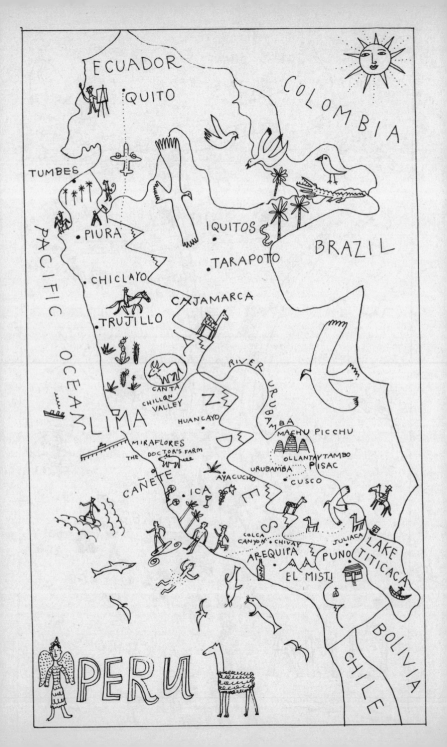

'Hold tight to the feather of your dreams
Lest the wind that brought it to your hands
Should blow it free again
High over the mountains
To the deserts of eternity.'

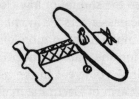

1

In the Beginning

The village of Brigue, Switzerland, valley of the Rhône, 23 September 1910. Twenty-three-year-old aviator Jorge Chávez, Paris-born of Peruvian parents, takes off in his single-engine, single-seater Blériot to attempt the first overflight of the Alps following the route of the Simplon Pass towards Milan, a distance of some seventy-five miles.

'Whatever happens,' he proclaims boldly, 'I shall be found on the other side of the mountains.'

So saying, he gives a nonchalant wave of farewell in the manner of the day. And, defying the pessimistic pundits, he is right. The challenge presented by the spectacular snow-capped peaks is brushed aside. Unfortunately, as the triumphant pilot comes in to land, the wings of his fragile plane crumple with fatigue. Jorge falls to the ground and never speaks again, dying four days later.

The city of Lima, Peru, valley of the River Rimac, 14 May 1999. It is nearly ninety years later that my routine, four-engined, two hundred and something-seater in-bound flight from Miami emerges from the shroud of low cloud to land at Jorge Chávez Airport. The passengers are intent on negotiating their way past the unsmiling immigration officials and no one spares a thought for the gallant magnificence of aviation history or for the irony inherent in the name of the airport. Plucked by the long arm of electronic mail from my involvement in not dissimilar activities in Central America, I have just one bag, enough to last me through my six-week assignment in South America. It has not been far to travel – southwards from inside the Tropic of Cancer, passing high over the Equator, and then earthwards, coming to rest well north of the Tropic of Capricorn – and I feel that the change in scenery from hospital management consultancy in Belize to the role of health centre adviser in Peru (albeit conspicuously unspecified and wanting for terms of reference) should not prove too traumatic. Assuming, of course, that the gulf between the undefined invitation and reality is not too wide.

I run the gauntlet of the stone-faced customs officers, to be greeted considerably more warmly by the owners of the newly constructed private clinic that I am to assist in 'commissioning and opening', Dr Hermogenes Abelardo Abasalon and his wife, La Señora Coraima Pandora del Teodosia Zapallo-Chupado Palermo Bonomini. I have never met anyone before with such a long name.

'We like to have you here very well nice,' La Señora tells me breathlessly. 'Oh, is it bad said, please?'

'No. It's beautiful. Thank you.'

Leaving the air-conditioned cocoon of the airport buildings, we proceed through the dank autumnal chill of late-night Lima to the orange glow of the neon-lit car park. The eminent Doctor helps me with my battered suitcase, the magic carpet of my life, veteran of a hundred similar adventures, held together with rope and colourful labels, legacies of countless journeys into the unknown. We climb aboard the Doctor's equally battered, big, once-white truck and sit three abreast across the front. It is past midnight and serious viewing of the presently sleepy and subdued city of the conquistadors, founded in 1535, must wait until another day. Some eight million people on a site with more than two thousand years of history; but for the moment it is simply a matter of fleeting first impressions in the dark.

The Doctor and La Señora indicate items of possible interest as we drive across town to the distant district of Miraflores, sharing the road with the ubiquitous 'combi' mini-buses and the unsleeping Tico taxis, both of which proliferate in the pollution-laden downtown atmosphere. As a last-resort method of transportation, I am informed, the Ticos are nearly as cheap as the combis, have marginally fewer collisions, but possess a tendency to break in two when under stress. Like amoebae.

'Here in Lima we have the best qualified *taxistas* in the world. Just give them a fare of a few nuevos soles and they can ride you all around the city,' says Dr Hermogenes. 'Our taxi drivers do not always know where they are going but that is not the point. They are highly qualified accountants, engineers, executives, professors of medicine, architects and so forth. It is the economical condition of the country.'

The condition of the traffic, like the economy, is chaotic. We cross an intersection where the situation is doubly chaotic.

'Who has the right of way here?' I enquire, curious as to our immediate future.

'Well, it depends on the education of each one,' explains the Doctor calmly, as he spins the steering wheel right and left.

I remark on the numerous banks that we are passing, barred and closed because of the hour but nonetheless guarded by flak-jacketed police, heavily armed with automatic hand guns, rifles and shotguns. There's a message there. Or maybe several. Norbank, Citibank, Interbank, Banco República, Banco

Sudamericano, Banco Wiese, Banco Latino, Banco Sur, Banco del País, Banco Financiero, Banco del Trabajo, Banco de Progreso, Banco de la Nación, Banco del Nuevo Mundo, Banco de Lima Sudameris, Banco de Credito, Banco Banex, Banco Continental, Banco Santander Central Hispano, the banking names flow and flow like the outpourings of an incontinent cashpoint. More messages.

'I don't know why we have so many banks in Peru,' reflects La Señora. 'Nobody has any money. And that is the Palace of Justice,' she adds wistfully, pointing out a grandly illuminated neo-classical building. 'It doesn't work. We don't have any justice either.'

We note another landmark. 'This is my old school,' continues my guide. 'Not too many people can get in there. One day they call me. "Señora Coraima," they say, "we need you. Your help and your artistic influence." "Wait for me," I say. "I am coming." I promise, but I don't know if I do it. I was very proud to went to school there. When I left I gave a speech out of the top of my head.'

As we pass a glittering shopping mall, the Doctor recalls that in his younger days everything on sale seemed to come from Gran Bretaña, from toys to toffees, trousers and tricycles to tractors. 'Now everything comes from the other direction,' he muses resignedly, 'including our President.'

I admire the fine trees in the parks, half-visible in the gloom. There is also sufficient light to contemplate the Amazonic curves of the cloned look-alike traffic police women mounted diminutively astride their gleaming Harley Davidsons.

'They are plastic,' remarks the Doctor, presumably meaning the trees. 'Here we have no rain.'

This is half true: there is hardly any serious rain in cloudy Lima, just a little *garua* drizzle in the winter. Lima la Gris, Lima the Grey. If by chance there is a shower in the city, then you can read about it on the front page of the newspaper the following morning. Those *Limeños* old enough to remember still talk about the day in 1970 when it rained for several hours and the streets flooded. I glance at the Doctor but he is concentrating on the road. How such magnificent trees grow is a mystery. La Señora senses my perplexity.

'Yes, these are fine trees,' she tells me. 'It's such a pity we don't have rain. Lima is not so much of a rainy place, more of a desert. But these are special trees not to die.'

I am duly installed in my new home, blinking at the sumptuousness of the gleaming four-storeyed, white-fronted Clinic, created by La Señora the artist for her husband the distinguished Doctor, which seems to be nearly as grand as the Palace of Justice although on a slightly smaller scale. Different in style too, with skilfully blended eclectic English architectural undertones, Georgian bow-fronted windows on the ground floor surmounted by balustraded Regency balconies on the second. And it works too, or at least, it should shortly.

'Our Clinic is mainly for the expecting woman,' explains La Señora.

As it is late, we enter through the darkness of the side door. The Doctor is reassuring.

'This is the back door,' he tells me, 'but don't worry, it is the same house.' Then he indicates a hosepipe tap protruding from the wall. 'Please mind the faucet,' comes the advice. 'Unless you are careful it can catch you in different parts.'

The Doctor is right, it can. In the coming days I am forcibly reminded of his caution on more than one occasion. However, for the moment we are proceeding ever upwards.

'Your bedroom is not in the attic,' says La Señora, reading my thoughts, 'but it is on the fourth floor which is the top. We do not have the lift yet. Or a fire escape.' Then, as though to distract my attention from the absence of both the former and particularly the latter, she explains somewhat rapidly that the operating theatre, tea-room and pharmacy are on the first floor, the consulting rooms and patients' waiting area are on the second, the suites for overnight patients, the laboratory and the gymnasium-cum-lecture hall are on the third, and, finally, that sundry offices, the laundry and various store-rooms are my companions on the fourth floor and that there are startlingly but conveniently at least a dozen bathrooms on hand throughout the building.

We ascend the ultimate flight of stairs to arrive out of breath at my room and I am grateful that I brought only the one suitcase. La Señora proudly throws open the door. Another explanation. 'The style is perhaps as a ship's cabin, which you may like as I know that once upon a time you were a sailor, and if you want, when you are resting in bed you may reach out and hold on to both sides of your room at the same time. Just inform me if you would like a hole cut in the ceiling so that you can see the sky passing by, the birds flying and watch the silent stars. Also from your bed you can look out across this interesting internal balcony which I myself designed and you may note what is happening in our auditorium on the third floor just below.'

And vice versa, I reflect, for those in the finely panelled lecture room with its striking, exquisitely fashioned pale flooring.

'This unique and striking wood I imported from Scandinavia,' says La Señora, following not only my gaze but my thoughts. 'It is true that the Amazon rainforest is closer but it is imperilled.'

Very soon, in a matter of weeks, the Clinic will dispense obstetric and gynaecological care, these being the specialities of the exceptional and nationally renowned Dr Hermogenes, highly qualified alumnus of the Johns Hopkins University Hospital, Baltimore. Building of The Ladies' Healthcare Clinic is almost complete, and shortly the euphoniously named, stalwart, raggedy team of Lupi Pancho the deranged electrician, Leonardo da Painter, Koki, Demaisio and Huaranga, shiftily overseen by Portencio and equally shady Hortencio, will be off to mix cement, join wires, connect pipes, lay bricks, grout tiles, cut wood and slap paint and plaster on someone else's surfaces. And hopefully their place will be taken by a rich and bountiful harvest of roundly pregnant ladies interspersed by the wishful and the wistful. Indeed, we are all full of hope.

To assist the process, La Señora embarks on a touch of creative marketing. She passes word that a wealthy member of the British aristocracy has arrived to assist in the launch of her new project. The effect of this fantasy is immediate. The Clinic is graced with a steady stream of ladies of a certain age, curious to meet this imagined addition to Lima high society. La Señora is similarly graciously pleased to receive them. Afternoon tea becomes an imported feature of the daily programme.

'*¡Qué linda!*' trill the visiting ladies, richly bejewelled and immaculately clad for the occasion. 'How beautiful! *¡Preciosa!* Maybe we can have a tea cup together this afternoon?'

Everybody loves our Clinic, especially the Victorian tearoom with its English cottage-garden flowery wallpaper, the delicate bone china, the silver cream jugs, shiny sugar bowls and tiny tongs, the doll's house tables and slender chairs. La Señora passes the miniature ginger biscuits and pours the tea.

'Is there sugar inside the tea?' enquire the visitors, huge pearls a-quiver on befreckled bosoms.

'No. One lump or two?'

The freshly sweetened ladies edge towards the subject uppermost in their thoughts.

'Is the good Lord with you today?' they enquire in a careless, offhand manner.

'*Sí*,' replies La Señora solemnly. 'The Lord is with us.' She pauses for effect.

'And is the good Lord well?'

'*Sí*, the Lord is well. He has a little age, but he is very fit.'

Afterwards La Señora tells me, 'I am saying you are too much fit, I think I put too many flowers on your head and I am doing too much publicity for you.' But for the time being the ladies digest this information together with their ginger nuts. Overall they decide that the news is satisfactory.

'*¡Qué bueno!* Great! Where did you find him?'

'I met him at the airport.'

'You found him at the airport?'

'Yes, I carried him here in a golden chair. But at the beginning I asked to myself, "What can I do to get a British man?" Then I just wrote to London and said please send me one British man, airmail. Then London asked me for further details, because that's the way they are there. So I answered them that I need a British man urgent. Please send him here to Lima.'

'And they sent you the good Lord?'

La Señora inclines her head. After all, how can an inclination of the head be an untruth?

'Now England has lost some of the jewellery in the crown.'

'*¡Qué bueno!* And will the good Lord be taking tea?'

'Possibly, but I do believe he is watering the garden,' says La Señora, sipping from her Earl Grey and not forgetting the lofted little finger.

'Watering the garden!' exclaim the visiting ladies, somewhat surprised. This is not normally seen as an aristocratic occupation in Peru.

'The good Lord loves all things, especially Nature's flowers,' comes the swift explanation.

'Ah!' sigh the ladies. '*Claro que sí*.' Yes, indeed.

Long may the myth prevail. It is excellent for business. Time, tides and profligate bank loans wait for no man.

*

As it happens, La Señora herself is not bereft of noble, indeed regal connections. Not, as might be imagined, of Inca or Chimu lineage, but Swedish. Which helps yet further to explain the origin of those previously remarked beautifully laid and sanded, time and money consuming auditorium floorboards.

'It is good to have blue blood,' she informs us, 'but even better to have a nobleness of spirit, an aristocracy of the soul. For the poor in spirit are poor in everything. It is a gypsy thought. The class comes from the crib. Here we have at least two Perus, probably more. Yes, the same thing occurs in England. Know that I am also of Swedish nobility. Now perhaps you are wondering how was my great-grandfather? Well, I never met him in fact.'

Documents, leather-bound books of reference and coats of arms are produced for the enlightenment of anyone who mischances to express interest in the subject. This is not all, although the precise details are rather more hazy. At times the name of Bismarck drops casually into the conversation, generally later in the evening rather than earlier. Even the Bourbons are mentioned. On other occasions we are transported to Arabia, with shadowy hints of dark Bedouin princes with far-horizon eyes and hawk noses, lounging by lamplight in richly carpeted tents fragrant with incense, heavy with romance and intrigue. Whilst outside in the starlit desert night, camels, those noble ships of the sands, fart restively in their sleep. No one can fail to be captivated by the vision and spellbound we listen.

'Royalty? Oh, you just grow with it,' declares La Señora easily.

Certainly, and it has to be said, she has never once been seen watering the garden.

The blessings of birth and royal lineage aside, there is still much to be done in the Clinic: functional and important medical trappings to be procured, unfunctional and extravagantly unnecessary furniture to be installed, sensuously thick carpets to be laid, brocaded calming curtains of immense weight to be hung. At every turn, the walls are decorated with gilt-framed paintings from the brush of La Señora herself, gifted as she is with an appropriate penchant for depicting the disrobed female form. Everything for La Señora's baby, the Clinic, is to be not only perfect but perfectly tasteful. So we set to and roll up our sleeves, metaphorically at least. There are loyal staff to be recruited, prosaic policies and procedures to be agreed and inscribed.

One of the first priorities is to make ready twin consulting rooms for her husband, the in-demand Doctor, so that he may attend two patients almost simultaneously in the manner pioneered by ancient Egyptian dentists with four arms. The expectant operating theatre must wait awhile, vital equipment is pending, delayed by customs processes, paperwork and those all-important Peruvian 'facilitating payments' that have similarly hampered installation of the ultrasound machine. Likewise the pharmacy and the laboratory must take their turn and are relegated to the waiting list. But we need staff immediately, so a list of essential personnel is made and then promptly halved. More people, more problems. More pay, too.

'I shall contact Abraham for the cleaning,' states La Señora.

'Abraham?' As usual my mind takes the wrong path.

'He has worked excellently for my family for many years on and on. When he is off he washes cars in the *plaza*.'

Good, Abraham it is, leaving one nurse, one cashier and one administrator; that will do nicely. Advertisements are placed in *El Comercio*, the response is immediate. Regardless of the official figures, unemployment, under-employment or mis-employment is running at over fifty per cent in the city of Lima. Some say the figure is eighty per cent. The mounds of applications are sifted, selections are made for interviews, the British adviser is co-opted to the board. When La Señora tells the applicants that they will work from eight in the morning to nine at night for the equivalent of one or two hundred pounds a month, nobody in the room blinks except me. On Saturdays we will try to finish at two in the afternoon, she concludes brightly, and thus the process of staff selection is completed.

'There,' declares La Señora decisively, briskly overruling the alternative findings of the panel. 'Dulce shall be our nurse and Ernestina will do the money. But who will do the papers? I think Señorita Hilda will be that person. She has a moustache but she will be strict and efficient.'

'Couldn't we give Miss Afrodita a try?' I venture, for no good reason other than the obvious charm of her scenic virtues.

La Señora looks at me sharply but acquiesces. It is early days. 'Yes,' she says, 'you may try.'

But on the following Monday morning there is no Afrodita at the door so we have to settle for heavily hirsute Hilda and I am left to reflect on the paradoxes and perversities of personnel planning. At least we have diminutive Dulce and bespectacled Ernestina.

'It is for the best,' observes La Señora, straightening the self-satisfied pencils on her desk with an air of finality.

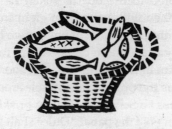

2

Morro Solar

The weekend, although abbreviated, is upon us. Activity in the opulent ambience of The Ladies' Healthcare Clinic ceases briefly in favour of sight-seeing. In Lima the choices are many. Perhaps we will start where Francisco Pizarro founded the city: the Plaza Mayor contains the Presidential Palace, the Archbishop's Palace and the grand Cathedral where the official guide informs visitors: 'Don Francisco Pizarro is dead here. His bones are in these boxes.' Perhaps we will start behind the *plaza* in the stately Desamparados railway station or maybe in the picturesque post office, La Casa de Correos y Telégrafos, with its impressively ornate arcade. Perhaps we will undertake a tour of the intricately carved antique balconies of Lima or visit the church of San Francisco with its corpse-filled catacombs. We may go to the once acclaimed Museo de Oro del Perú with its now allegedly fraudulent exhibits of non-Inca treasure, and then advance to the waiting delights of the shamelessly acrobatic erotic pottery gathering dust in the Museo Arqueológico Rafael Larco Herrara. Or possibly we will find our way to the overlooked Museo Pedro D. Osma in the artistic district of Barranco with its incomparable collection of paintings of the Cusqueña school and other surprises, such as a Tampion longcase clock.

In the event, for my touristic initiation La Señora opts for the fish market. She has been seized with an unstoppable desire to procure a cornucopia of *pescados y mariscos* for an extravagant seafood lunch beyond compare.

Just along the coast from the Lima fish market lies Morro Solar, unaccountably omitted from the majority of the guide books. Unaccountable because with only a little stretch of the imagination it could be said that Morro Solar is to Lima as Pão de Azúcar is to Rio de Janeiro. Sugar Loaf looks down on Copacabana; Morro Solar oversees Horseshoe Bay and the Costa Verde. At this point it is best for the imagination to stop stretching, quite apart from the fact that the Costa is not so Verde these days. The moisture that used to exude from the cliff face to provide life for the green vegetation has largely been diverted by various building projects and other so-called developments with the result that much of the cliffs has reverted to a sad sandy brown. Restoration is reputedly in hand, of course.

Anyway, we take the coast road and head for the fish market. The Pacific rollers en route are dotted with the heads of surfers looking like so many seals as they wait for the right moment to practise their graceful art. An atlas is needed, but it seems possible that those giant leisurely waves have rolled lazily all the way from Tahiti.

Buying fish in the slippery bustle of the smelly market is also an art. For La Señora, that is. Whilst she revels in risqué repartee with the vendors, *las pescaderas*, stocky ladies with fat shiny aprons, red hands and sharp filleting knives, I confine myself to marvelling at the quantity and colourful variety of the unfamiliar fish arrayed on the wet stone stall slabs, feeling a bit like one of the patient pelicans sitting in watchful rows on the quayside.

'See the fishermans?' asks La Señora, taking time off from inspecting the brightness of eye and sanguineous sparkle of the inner gills of her prospective purchases. 'We have a lot of fish. My affinity is with the ocean.' As well it might be with a larder as huge as the Pacific Ocean on the doorstep providing such bounty day in, day out, year after year, up and down the coast. (Although the time will surely come when even the Pacific reveals itself to have limits. Genesis will be defied and the great waters will no more 'bring forth abundantly the moving creature that hath life'.) But La Señora never does things by halves. Her plump and fleshy selections, *corvina*, *lenguado*, assorted shellfish, boxes and bags enough to last for several months, all are loaded and the car sinks visibly.

The ascent to Morro Solar is steep, but the view along the coast and out to sea is magnificent. As we drive past the barrier at the foot of the access road the *watchiman* makes that peculiarly Peruvian sign of two splayed fingers in front of the eyes.

'Look at what?' I ask.

However, we are left wondering. But not for too long.

There is a giant illuminated cross at the highest point of the cliff, while a little way below is a monument in memory of Peruvians who fell during the disastrous 'Pacific War' with Chile, 1879–1883. We join a group of schoolchildren and their teachers to read the inscription, and in the process of trying to picture the events of those dark days just over a century ago I am suddenly jerked back to the present by La Señora's urgent voice.

'Run, Señor John! Run!'

Run? Why? I look round. The children and their teachers have drifted away and are about a hundred metres distant. We are isolated, except that we are rapidly being joined by a gang of five evil ruffians appearing from behind the low wall surrounding the car park. Problems. La Señora is running like a lizard towards the safety of the school party, going well. Poetry in motion indeed. I am slow out of the blocks, but I get the message and follow suit confidently. But my best is not good enough. Disappointing really. Too many marathons must have knocked the edge off my speed. It is like a rugby football nightmare, legs pumping and going for the corner flag for a certain try, only to find that somehow the entire opposing team have reached the line first and closed the gap. I fail to make ground on La Señora, but the same could not be said of the opposition. They have it all worked out and encircle us neatly, silently, just the scuff of hard-working boots.

We break the silence to call after the school group.

'Help! Help us please!'

They turn, stare curiously, and turn back. That's the way it is in the modern world. La Señora comes to a halt, she is puffed out. Perhaps she had gone out too fast. I come to a halt. No doubt about it, I had gone out too slowly. We are caught, arms pinned behind us. They are an unappealing-looking bunch, our assailants, but I doubt that I could readily recognize any of them again. I have a momentary vision of launching an amazing kung fu (or something) assault on them. *Aaaargh, kick, twist, back flip. Pow! Bam! Aaaargh again, another Kapow, feint left, feint right, reverse kick, forward thrust, double loop with tuck. Three men down. The cowardly remainder running for safety.*

'*¡Hijos de putas!' I shout after them.*

La Señora embraces me, the hero of the hour. We step over the prostrate bodies and stroll back to the car, hand in hand.

But it doesn't happen like that. Kung fu is not in my repertoire. I hesitate for a moment and the gang leader reaches into his pocket to produce a bulge that could have been a pistol, or a knife or maybe just a nice weighty club. Certainly not a packet of Polo mints. That settles it. It's my move. I twist sufficiently and manage to reach into my pocket. I produce the contents, nearly 200 dollars. Rats. That was my subscription for the gymnasium. And recent events have just indicated that I could use the training. I feel a bit depressed the way things are turning out, but the ugly hoods seem quite pleased. They have more than enough for a few fixes or a bottle or two of pop, depending on their predilections. They exchange glances, we are released and off they go, back over the wall.

What you might call a minimalistic mugging. Limited display of emotion by either side. No dialogue. Although in subsequent accounts La Señora insists that I threw my hands in the air with the words 'Take everything I have!' She is an artist, you see. Artists live by their imagination. Come to think of it, I am sure I heard her say to the muggers, 'Leave me alone, he's the one with the money!' But of course, I've never mentioned it to her and anyway, this is not the moment for recriminations.

We head back to the car, some fifty metres away. In the circumstances it somehow seems appropriate to jog. Oh, well, I tell myself stoically, we broke the rules, dropped our guard and paid the price. No broken bones, just a little bruised pride. And, of course, pity about my gymnasium subscription. I might be tempted to take up kung fu.

'¡*Caracho!*' exclaims La Señora. 'They are coming back!'

Caracho indeed. Veteran of at least half a dozen assorted attacks in Lima, she knows the form. The gang can scent rich pickings in the car: a handbag, camera, credit cards. ¡*Dios mío!* Now we really do have problems. We break into a run, but the thugs are between us and our means of escape.

'The Clinic staff salaries are in the boot,' pants La Señora.

Dios mío again. And the fish. Now things really are getting depressing.

And then, when all seems lost, a small miracle occurs, right there at Morro Solar. It's a big miracle actually. Over the brow of the hill and into the deserted car park bounces a funny little van, straight out of a Disney cartoon, its body too big for its wheels. Smiling driver, big wagging golden Labrador, little boy, also smiling.

'I know him, I know him!' cries La Señora. 'He's our vet!'

She does and he is. We jump in to safety. The wolves slide back over the wall, sulky and thwarted. Except for one, clearly the creative member of the gang, who stands his ground and suddenly engages in furious arm circling, pretending to be a fitness fanatic sampling the morning freshness.

But it's all over. Hurried explanations, a fraction excited and slightly breathless, we regain our car (and the salaries and the fish) and down the hill we go in convoy. We wave our saviours goodbye. They wave back, still smiling and wagging.

'I suppose we should go and report it to the police,' I suggest.

'Report what?' La Señora stares at me. 'Are you *loco*?' She explains what may be best termed the 'cultural aspects' of my suggestion. It is my turn to stare.

'Well, maybe there is an emergency number we could ring?'

'There is,' says La Señora, 'but I can't remember it and anyway nobody uses it.'

'Why not?' I ask, suspiciously. Normally La Señora has an encyclopaedic memory for telephone numbers.

'Nobody answers,' comes the swift retort.

I run out of bright ideas.

'Don't worry,' says La Señora consolingly, 'I'll ring the Mayor.'

And she does, she rings the Mayor there and then to express her total dissatisfaction with the morning's events. No problem remembering his number. These days the citizens of the global village wear their mobile telephones like an article of clothing. For Peruvians the relationship seems to be particularly intimate: the beloved 'cellular' is one of the three things they like to have next to their skin.

The call to the Mayor completed, we look at each other. Time for lunch at Casa Bonomini. All that fresh air and exercise seems to have given us quite an appetite. And as it happens, we still have a boot full of fresh fish.

A few weeks later we read in the newspaper that our gang of muggers have grown overconfident and have been caught by the police after robbing a group of Japanese tourists. But tragically, a month or so afterwards we receive the very sad news that our Good Samaritan the vet has been knocked down late one night and killed at the roadside on the way to his home while changing the wheel of his Disneyland car.

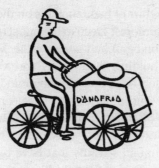

3

Miraflores

'Look at the flowers' – the aptly named up-market Limeño district of Miraflores, now my adopted home as the original six-week term of my stay has somehow become indefinite. Miraflores: location of our burgeoning Clinic and also home to many of our clients, where some of the houses are so large that they have separate numbers for the garages. In case anyone should want to send a letter to the *chofer*. A proverbial profusion of colour: bougainvillea of all shades of red and purple tumbling over the high protective walls of the secluded villas; blue jacaranda, yellow-flowering *guarango* trees, orange *tulipana africana* lining the avenues fringed with freshly laundered lawns; lantana, canna lilies, hibiscus, oleander, multicoloured geraniums of course, immense hollyhocks of unimagined grandeur and even roses grace the carefully tended gardens. In the parks, sweetly scented, giant, rustling eucalyptus, monkey puzzles, flame of the forest and pine trees, home to so many birds that birdsong rather than the noise of traffic is the predominant sound first thing in the morning, in the evening and in the quiet of the weekend.

Birdsong and the whirr of hand mowers on the manicured grass that is a startling rainforest green in the midst of the desert that is Lima, with the choreographed *jardineros*, the scarcely paid gardeners, vacantly holding their hoses and watering the road instead of the borders on account of their minds being elsewhere or nowhere. Migrating *jardineros* who have come down from the high Andes by the thousand to make their fortune in the big city, following faint tracks and rock-strewn paths running alongside the cascading mountain streams that have been similarly harnessed to serve the needs of thirsty Lima, the very contents of which are now being squandered with absent-minded abandon.

And on the leafy pavements of Miraflores, a greater number of perambulating nannies, neatly uniformed in blue or pink with white lace, than might have been found on an English promenade at the turn of the previous century. Pushing highly-sprung baby carriages that more than likely have close connections with Dr Hermogenes, or assisting their elderly charges, watched lasciviously by the indolent, somnolent security guards supposedly overseeing the grand houses. The yellow-jacketed D'Onofrio ice cream sellers, *los heladeros*, pedal their hopeful yellow tricycles to and fro. Blowing shrill, irritating toy *trompetas* or *cornetitas* to advertise their presence and sharing the road with other occasional vendors: purveyors of jumbo-sized potted palms and priapic cacti, colourful cartloads of brushes and brooms, flat-topped barrows with wooden wheels and iron rims that grate on the concrete, laden with fruit and vegetables. La Señora especially favours the latter, suppliers to her household for countless years.

'Here you see, this is wonderful Peru,' she explains. 'The fruit and vegetable man just comes, you take everything you need and you pay him next week.' I half expect to see her 'By Appointment' crest on the side of the barrow. 'In your country even one potato is expensive. And also, sometimes these fruits they fell to the floor by themselves, so they are not raised hurry-up.'

Yes, wonderful Peru. *El frutero* has an indecipherable notebook for his grubby accounts, regularly baptized in dirty bath-water or stale tea, and he is pleased to charge the first figure that comes into his inventive head. But his produce is beyond compare: exotic white-fleshed chirimoya fruits, ripe mangoes, lucuma, abounding bananas, oranges, mandarins, apples, avocados, ciruelos like juicy red plums, granadillas, grenadines, yellow and purple striped pepinos, trellises of grapes, pert little lemons and bursting great melons. The variety seems endless.

La Señora is less pleased with the ubiquitous ice cream sellers. Those ever-optimistic, proliferating yellow tricycles, she says, should have a compulsory family-planning programme, to be shared with Lima's combis and Ticos.

'This blowing-hooting is an *escándalo*,' she declares. 'I am not an old person, I am a tempered person, but it is too much.'

La Señora prefers the *afilador de cuchillos*, the knife sharpener, the mender of pots and pans, wheeling his ancient wooden handcart. Jilguero she calls him, the goldfinch, because his reedy pipes resemble the song of the bird of that name. Revolución Caliente, the 'hot revolution' ginger biscuit man, is also a favourite, doing his rounds with a high-pitched call and lantern. But he appears to be the last of the line. Maybe soon, like Jorge Chávez, Revolución Caliente will be no more.

In the late evening come the supper sellers with their *tambores*, drumming away to draw our attention to their chicken-or-pork-with-corn-in-a-banana-leaf *tamales*, their rice and chicken or iguana *juanes*, similarly wrapped, or their *humitas* of sweetcorn in a corn leaf. La Señora invariably answers the call of the drums and we eat well, especially skinny Ernestina, our careless cashier seated comfortably in the seclusion of her office under the stairs, dropping crumbs into the accounts as she feeds her youthful desires so that the grease spots look like extra noughts and we have trouble balancing the books. Enigmatic Ernestina, hidden under the stairs, hiding her secret lives behind solemn horn spectacles as

21

she scribes the ledgers in cheerful manuscript and dreams of computerization and other things.

My airy office, situated on the heights of the top floor of the Clinic, is neighbour to the eyrie that contains my ever-welcoming bed. The very minimum of commuting to be done but nonetheless my time-keeping must be rigid. It doesn't do for sternly serious Señorita Hilda – she of the lightly sleeping though darkly veiled appetites, undefined and unknown especially to herself – to surprise me toying with an eight o'clock bowl of cornflakes on my desk when the sun is already high and the business of the day is pressing.

The wide office window overlooks the garden, which is really the car park for the growing flow of our fashionable patients. How is it that the dear immaculately coiffured ladies manage to hit so many of my pots and run over so many of my plants as they inexpertly manoeuvre and finally park their gleaming cars? They must be preoccupied. They are about to be seen by the Doctor; their minds are on other things. In a world wherein both a hair appointment and a visit to the dress-maker's boutique are unavoidable precursors to a medical appointment, life is surely stressfully complex.

However, countering the increasing daily depredations of the visiting stream, the Lima climate is humid, gentle and healing. In the courtyard I have brazen marigolds, gay petunias, mini-ature palms, morning glory, evening star, pastel blue and yellow daisies, vivid lobelia to match the sky, vulgar nasturtiums, prickly cactus and much more, all in spite of those preoccupied patients randomly coming and going for half the day.

In our Clinic, as in Life, presentation is everything and I have expanded my non-existent terms of reference to include care of the garden. Nonetheless, perhaps it would be better to admit defeat and to invest in a mountain *jardinero* like everyone else. Except that gardening is such an intensely intimate and personal activity; as in marriage, contracting out or delegating the detailed responsibilities can never be entirely satisfactory. Thus it is that of an afternoon or in the supposed solitude of the Sabbath I am to be found in the courtyard of the Clinic, tenderly nursing my charges, trowel and secateurs in hand, surprised at intervals by the purring arrival of yet another gleaming Mercedes or Porsche, the incumbents of which sweep past without even so much as a cursory nod in the direction of my humbly kneeling form. 'The rich man in his castle, the poor man at his gate'; gardening is indeed 'a renunciation of worldly ambition'. Anyway, everybody needs a hobby, even if only to fill the day.

La Señora is a proud member of the British Royal Horticultural Society. She claims, probably with good reason, to be one of the very few members in the entire continent of South America. Moreover, she tells us that she was at one time President not only of the Programa de Investigación y Producción de Hortalizas Exóticas of Huachipa but also of the Centro de Investigación y Producción de Endivias de Bruselas 'Witloof', similarly of Huachipa (both now defunct). Both individually and collectively these obscure horticultural honours clearly entitle her to make provocatively dismissive assessments concerning the progress of the Clinic garden.

'In Lima, geraniums are weeds. Permit me to tell you this.'

'Oh. Sorry.'

Or to apply her own artistic criteria.

'One pot, one colour. Please follow this rule.'

'Oh.'

Or to take unilateral action when deemed necessary.

'This plant encourages *serpientes*, I have pulled it out.'

Snakes? Snakes alive. I slither off in sulky silence. In life, every day is a day of learning.

It has to be said that La Señora's own garden is devoid of flowers. Not a sausage. Envy is a terrible thing. And not content with this, she has one more parting shot as I take my offended leave of her.

'Not only the Royal Horticultural Society,' she calls after me. 'I am many other things. For example, I am a member of The Women's Prostitution Group of Peru.'

Jiminy cricket! Every day is indeed a day of learning. And it is as well to remember that at times translation between languages can be an inexact science.

The gardens either side of mine have inviting swimming pools, patiently waiting for the Lima fog to clear. And it does, some days, though mainly in the summer months December to April, when the temperature climbs from the sixties, through the seventies to the high eighties. Then it will be my turn to wait patiently, for the invitations to swim which never come.

The garden beyond the Clinic has a large tree, dead now but still home to countless doves and pigeons. Happy birds, they coo contentedly and copulate all day long. Perhaps there are worse formulae for life. The pots under the tree have to be washed daily. Sometimes a pair of glorious red cardinals comes to share the dead tree, sometimes we are visited by anonymous yellow birds and chirpy blue birds and often by the tiny *picaflores*, the fluttering colibri. But it is the occasional screeching arrival of the green parrots that really disturbs the pigeons. Off they flutter, circling in confusion like elderly matrons caught in a sudden squall on a summer pier. The green parrot gang, undisciplined hooligans of the sky, laugh and mimic, and then suddenly fly off to torment and terrorize the occupants of some other tree in some other park, swooping and chattering high over the cluttered flat roofs of Lima in their distinctive flight.

Hospitable Casa Bonomini, home of the Doctor and La Señora and now my second home, is four blocks distant from the Clinic, just over the invisible border of Miraflores into the equally salubrious and leafy suburb of San Isidro. Within easy lunchtime and evening reach, it is also home for Medical

Student One and Medical Student Two, heirs of the Zapallo-Chupado Palermo Bonomini dynasty. They are at the age of invincibility and are as students are: generally inhabiting some other planet and only returning to Mother Earth when in need of food and sleep.

Indeed, Casa Bonomini is something of a menagerie. There are the pattering Yorkshire terriers, formerly ten but now eroded to three: Valentino, Pierre and Stephanie. Charm and promiscuity they have in equal measure whilst their indiscriminate, inconsiderate incontinence makes life in Casa Bonomini not without its hazards.

'I am sorry for this situation,' apologizes La Señora sadly and regularly. 'My floor is humbled now, my carpet it has been insulted again. I couldn't train the dogs. I couldn't even train my children.'

In uncharitable moments one is tempted to contemplate the possibility of further erosion.

'These dogs should pass to a better life,' says Medical Student One, broodingly.

But with their tiny pink tongues and dancing walk they are well practised in the art of seduction and survival, visiting *el salón de belleza* regularly to return fluffy and trimmed with bows on their heads.

'They just give the cold nose on my leg to remind me to put them to the bath,' says La Señora. 'If you wish, you may take these dogs for a ride.'

'For a walk?'

'If that's what you want.'

But the Doctor immediately advises against it. 'In Peru only a particular kind of person does that.'

'You mean . . . ?'

'Exactly.'

Carlotta *la tortuga* is another matter entirely: a highly refined tortoise of rare vivacity and natural dignity. Only a 'she' by presumption (it is hard to tell with tortoises), Carlotta, or perhaps Carlos, has a riveting turn of speed. At the sound of La Señora's voice she knows that with haste and good fortune she is in for a scratch and a tickle on the back of her scaly head, food and good conversation: all the essentials of carapacial contentment. Party-loving, ankle-nipping Carlotta will outlast us all.

Her best friend used to be Benito-the-Monkey ('He was the most happy monkey in this world'), but regrettably, even for Casa Bonomini, Benito's behaviour was too outrageous and he was donated to a zoo.

Charlie-the-Mouse should also be in a cage but has proved difficult to catch. He is but infrequently sighted in person, the only evidence being his teeth marks on any chocolate left unattended.

As La Señora explains, 'We think Charlie-the-Chocoholic he is occupating the stereo speakers.'

The unceasing ebb and flow of pets and mascots: at first La Señora's predilection for collecting 'all creatures great and small' passed me by and the subliminal implications escaped me. Then one day I found myself pondering my own place in the order of things.

Fidel Contreras, also of the menagerie and *jardinero extraordinario*, has the distinction of tending the flowerless garden of Casa Bonomini. Contreras is his real name; yes, Contreras by name, Contreras by nature. Fidel is seen as a humorous topical appendage. To give him his due, he is something of an unsung world record holder. Few other gardeners can have laboured for so long and produced so little. His favourite pastime is watering, standing perfectly still, wearing his vacant smile. Second best activity is pulling the hose from one side of the garden to the other, or through the house, preferably during lunchtime. Still smiling. Worst activity is cutting the grass with his hand mower. No smile. Most ingenious achievement is transporting the hand mower on his pushbike. That, and not watering the grass so that he doesn't have to cut it.

'He is the most lazy of men,' exclaims the lady of the house. 'He has been with me for eighteen years and really has never worked once. The only reason he comes is to collect his salary.'

Once a year, and once a year only, Fidel is fired with a burst of energy and launches a spirited crusade against the environment. In the early spring he cuts back all the garden shrubs and creepers, resolutely resisting all endeavours to introduce any colour to the garden. Except green, that is. Even Fidel hasn't worked out how to stop the troublesome ingress of green into a garden. But no doubt he is giving the problem considerable thought. The annual horticultural cull completed, Fidel reverts to semi-hibernation. Maybe he too was a tortoise in a previous life, but possibly without Carlotta's charm.

Not only has he never once in living memory planted anything himself, he thwarts everyone else's efforts to grow flowers.

'Fidel, please water the new flowers that I have planted.'

'*Sí, señor*.' But he doesn't, never ever. He watches them die. Not his responsibility, nothing to do with him.

'Fidel, have you watered the new flowers?'

'*Sí, señor*.' But he hasn't.

'Well, please do it again. And stop saying "*Sí, señor*"!'

'*Sí, señ*—' He stops. Clever man.

It's just as well that the barren garden of Casa Bonomini is across the invisible border into snooty San Isidro and not in floral Miraflores.

Somehow or other, the days in the Clinic tick away. For Dr Hermogenes, rising early, long and caring consultations are punctuated by important although unexplained absences, assuredly medical in nature. For the resident British adviser, a touch of supervision here, a soupçon of forward contemplation there, the elusive Spanish language, the Peruvian Castellano, to be mastered and always the enchantingly seductive garden with the brazen marigolds beckoning through the window. For La Señora, rising later, well, clearly there are many outside demands on her time.

To the toiling trio comprising impassively statuesque Señorita Hilda, passively curvaceous Nurse Dulce and rattlingly ravenous Ernestina the carefree cashier, falls the burden of administering and orchestrating the daily comings and goings of the patients, maintaining the backbone of the operation. Cheerfully united by the adversity of shared travail, eight until late, Mondays to Fridays, they join tired hands at the end of each long day and slip thankfully through the handsome front door, their three disparate silhouettes disappearing into the darkness of the night, bound for hidden destinations and destinies closed for ever from our gaze.

As foretold by La Señora, almost accurately, clinical activity invariably finishes at two or at three or maybe four on Saturday afternoons and then the whole weekend lies before us, with only a few inconsiderate stragglers presenting at the Clinic to pass the time on Sundays and disturb my echoingly solitary occupancy, akin to Charlie-the-Chocoholic in the stereo speakers.

The dull and lethargic Limeño winter gives way to spring with its flashes of sunshine and, appropriately in tune with the shift of the seasons, the warmly welcoming portals of The Ladies' Healthcare Clinic, Lima, open ever wider to greet our patients. We are making progress, even though the Bank, not unwisely (but quite unreasonably in our view), declines our request for a further extension of credit. We need to install an elevator to move in-patients from the ground-floor operating theatre to their upstairs rooms. No lift means no in-house deliveries, and we are limited to minor day-surgery.

This is but a temporary constraint and meantime we form a rewarding liaison with Dr Cleeber, the successful cosmetic cutter. He is pleased to have access to our excellent facilities and in no time at all is arcanely nipping and tucking, snipping and sucking behind the closed doors of the now briskly functioning operating room with the help of his anonymously masked team of assistants, reshaping discontented profiles, even if not remoulding discontented lives. Either way, the contribution to the Clinic coffers is welcome.

Chuckling Dr Ching joins the team, sanguine pathologist that he is, living proof of ancient and not-so-ancient trans-oceanic Asiatic intercontinental migratory patterns, smilingly transporting medical samples, swabs, smears and specimens to his laboratory in his all-purpose plastic lunch box for careful analysis.

Next, balding but youthful Dr Desastre, impecunious, unconventional master of avant-garde Spanish dietary advice, opportunely invests his last pesos in renting a Clinic consulting room and offers his newly qualified nutritional services to all comers. 'Eat as much as you like,' he tells his roly-poly patients, 'particularly potatoes. Except aubergines, red peppers and peanuts, of course.' Then, incredibly, a week later when the naked guinea pigs remount the shivering scales, pounds have been shed. Nobody knows how or why. Probably on account of guilt and confusion brought on by a plethoral plenitude of Peruvian *papas*.

Last and definitely least comes mournfully Germanic Dr Vonday. He shrewdly aligns himself to the Clinic as understudy to gynaecological Dr Hermogenes, but as yet is still waiting in the wings, yet to have greatness thrust upon him and yet to confront his first patient in the flesh. Pending the elusive moment, he is generally to be found sitting morosely in the Victorian tea-room in preference to the barren loneliness of his unfrequented

Sprechzimmer, his *consultorio*, lugubriously munching intermittent truffles, apologizing for the war and mentally rehearsing medical jokes with which he tries to divert and entertain the hardworking Dr Hermogenes. Unsuccessful in his jocular efforts, as in most things, Dr Vonday reverts to serious conversation.

'Von day,' he informs the Doctor earnestly, 'everything vill be fine.'

Whereupon Dr Hermogenes chokes on his truffle and laughs louder than he did at any of the medical jokes, leaving Dr Vonday to puzzle over the curious sense of humour possessed by foreigners.

Thus it is, with the captain and the crew in place, the noble enterprise is ready for the formal launch, like a stately ship poised on the slipway. Over the course of the preceding agreeably unhurried weeks the team has been formed and metaphorically bedded down, and no one feels the need to question the identity of who is in fact the real captain, or who indeed is the sleeping partner. The doctors themselves share the amicably admiring tie of having each surmounted the not insignificant hurdle of lengthy medical training; the youthful trinity of administration, nursing and accounting are bonded by the burden of their daily labours. In turn, the two interdependent groups are linked by mutually respectful curiosity, born not least of the belief that neither has the capacity to perform the demanding functions of the other. Underlying all and subject to the demands of his moonlighting car-washing in the nearby *plaza*, Abraham attends at the Clinic to dust, sweep and polish, while above and over all rests the omnipresent guiding hand of La Señora, at times in person, more often exercising influence from further afield, but invariably omniscient.

On the chosen evening, faced in the finely floored auditorium by a dutifully attentive invited audience of family, friends and Clinic supporters, the Minister of Health himself, acquaintance of La Señora, suavely obliges with the obligatory words of officialdom, whilst the heavenly blessing is performed by the 'priest of the bullfighters', acquaintance of the Doctor.

I wonder at the incongruity of this latter connection, particularly when the visiting clergyman appears to have some difficulty in selecting a passage suitable to the occasion from his well-thumbed Bible. Scrabbling through to the Book of Revelation to no avail, he returns to the opening pages in search of inspiration and eventually settles for a few carefully chosen verses from Genesis as providing the rightly blended message of a great Beginning, Creation, Life and Hope, sagaciously stopping before the plot thickens.

Then, as afterwards we all stroll down the tree-lined road to pass through the ever-open doors of Casa Bonomini for celebratory champagne and congratulatory caviar canapés on Fidel's drought-stricken lawn, it is my turn to receive a shaft of revelation and I am reminded yet again that everybody needs a hobby. Bulls! That's what it is with the Doctor. Great four-legged fighting bulls.

Consequently, when October comes and the season of *las corridas* starts, we lose no time in heading off into the mountains in the Doctor's big, once-white truck for the first of the regional bullfights. We tell ourselves unconvincingly that it is the moment for a well-earned day away from the Clinic, even though, well-earned or otherwise, we know that in reality it is not a day's truancy we can truly afford. The exorbitant rate of interest being charged on our borrowing means that our daily outpourings to the Bank are such that every morning when the Clinic is unlocked for business we are a thousand dollars further into the red. But this is Peru, so we ignore the semantics and the bothersome arithmetic and off we gaily go, abandoning Dr Vonday to his sad and solitary contemplation of the pastries and leaving him nominally in charge of nothing, destined to wait for ever in the wings.

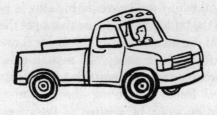

4

Feria Taurina de la Ciudad de Canta

We are late leaving the Clinic. It's normal but it means we will have to hurry if we are to arrive in Canta in time for the start of the bullfights. There are four of us. The Doctor behind the wheel of the big, once-white truck, La Señora, Aunt Hermenegilda and me. We sit squashed in a straight line, there is hardly space for the sandwiches, avocado and tomato with brown bread, but we manage. The Doctor drives with one arm on the window sill, cap tilted nonchalantly backwards as he changes gear continually and does battle with the Lima traffic. He controls our progress using that sixth sense known only to Limeño drivers, no quarter given or expected, an embargo on the use of the indicators in case anyone might reveal their intentions to the opposition. Use the horn instead; it makes more noise.

Progress is slow and sporadic, every second vehicle a passenger-laden combi belching noxious fumes, weaving from side to side, stopping and starting when least expected. La Señora sleeps, theatrically, to indicate displeasure with the general situation. But after half an hour and just in time before we all die from asphyxiation, or worse, we suddenly clear the seemingly endless city suburbs and find ourselves in the sunshine of the fertile Chillón valley.

To either side of us the down-at-heel sprawl of forlorn stores and dusty tenements with dirty curtains is miraculously replaced by fields of succulent leeks and fat cabbages, maize and fruit trees. Then come the mountains, barren and grey, containing gold and other minerals. It is well past two and the *Feria Taurina* starts at half past three, more or less. So we hurry on, the wide bonnet of the truck seeming to fill the narrow road so that I am grateful for the absence of anything travelling in the opposite direction. The Doctor is enjoying himself as he guides us one-handed through the twists and turns.

'Nice road for rallies,' he observes.

'Are you very rushed? No? Then don't overtake on this corner.'

This last comes from the sleeping Señora, accompanied by the faintest flicker of the eyelids. Magic. For a moment the Doctor is startled by this unexpected admonition, then he recovers his composure and back down goes his foot.

Occasional bridges are set at right angles to our line of advance. These present a special challenge for our driver. He accelerates as we approach and then flicks the truck sideways so that the tyres squeal. Fortunately his eye is good and we fly back and forth over the Río Chillón with a rumble of wheels and without mishap. My feet ache from pressing non-existent brakes and like the Doctor, I too have one hand out of the window. But mine grips the roof of the car with a fierce will for survival.

'We must be there soon,' I say hopefully.

'Only half the way,' replies the Doctor happily as we screech and thunder over another thin little bridge.

La Señora sleeps on. Aunt Hermenegilda chatters

contentedly. If you ever have the misfortune to be ship-wrecked, be sure to take a Peruvian with you. That way you will never run short of conversation.

Aunt Hermenegilda remembers travelling up this same road many years ago.

'My friends had a mine,' she remarks. 'Probably gold, but I forget now. We stayed there for five days. It was a wedding.' And as an afterthought she tells us, 'My brother also had a mine but he lost it.'

As you might lose a button from your coat, I suppose.

Then it is the Doctor's turn to reminisce. He recalls hurrying up this road long before the asphalt was laid, when it was just rocks and dust, bumps and potholes. The Land Rover he was in went slower and slower as the gradient increased but they made it, just in time for the opening ceremony. That night on the return journey the full extent of the problem became clear.

'Up the slopes the accelerator was sticking with no power,' explains the Doctor, 'down the slopes the car was running without the feet.'

Closer inspection revealed that the entire engine had broken free from its securing bolts and was sliding to and fro under the bonnet.

Suddenly a huge mining lorry appears and roars past in the opposite direction. There is scarcely room for us both. I look at the Doctor.

'That's why I hurry up,' he explains. 'In case we meet him on the bridge.'

As we approach 10,000 feet our own truck decides to become temperamental. The fertile fields have given way to cactus plants and little patches of grass on the mountainside for the occasional cow, and the air is markedly fresher. La Señora awakes.

'I have just woken up,' she remarks, to nobody in particular. 'I am perfectly fine.'

We are a long way from anywhere, not a house or human in

sight. But she needs to brush her hair. Immediately, now. Packed in as we are, finding the necessary bag and then the necessary comb is quite a major undertaking, interrupted by a gush of steam from under the bonnet.

'Ah, now the engine is a little warm,' says the Doctor, possibly slightly unnecessarily.

We stop. We need water for the radiator but the river now lies far below us in the valley bottom.

'The river is not so much,' Aunt Hermenegilda assures me. 'In the mountains it is not the raining time.'

So we drive on, slowly, until we reach a small spring that gurgles out from under the rocks by the roadside.

The ailing radiator is replenished and the smoke and steam clear in the breeze. We are almost within sight of Canta. Just a few hundred feet more. Climbing Everest must be like this. Then we discover the puncture.

'Now we are fried!' exclaims La Señora. 'The tyre is flatting!'

Fortunately it is only flatting at the bottom. We are anxious about the time, but not too much.

'He who is late, is late,' comes the philosophical observation from my companions.

Peruvians live in the belief that planes, trains and bullfights will always await their arrival if by any mishap they might be a fraction behind the clock.

La Señora, lifetime lover of toys and gadgets, forgets about finding her comb and produces from nowhere a magical little pump that comes to life when connected to the motor battery. It sets about its work and dances merrily on the tarmac as it pushes air back into the sick tyre. We climb on board and limp up to Canta. I wonder what miracle of foresight made La Señora bring that brave little pump.

The main street is thronged with excited townspeople, visitors and vendors. The magnificent toreadors pass by in a pick-up in full regalia. The Doctor, official *asesor taurino* for the great occasion, is much in demand, greeting old acquaintances.

We have to hurry a little, hearts beating loudly because of the altitude, but a modest fee of eight nuevos soles apiece sees us safely inside the *plaza* and precariously installed on the top plank of the seating. The grand entrance of the participants, colourfully adorned, is heralded by the band two paces to our right. The arena is packed, and more.

The big sign on the hoarding says *Plaza Portátil*.

'This is a moving bull ring,' Aunt Hermenegilda explains.

Not too much, I hope, and I worry about the strength of the scaffolding supporting our plank. Looking up the surrounding mountainsides I see scores of spectators saving themselves such anxieties and the price of a ticket.

The first bull is reluctant to join the fray and finally enters the *plaza* rump first. He need not have worried too much. The opening matador, or torero, is scarcely five feet tall and new to the game. He makes a succession of inept passes and then gestures extravagantly to the crowd, hips thrust forward, shoulders back, head proudly tilted, the graceful curve of the upflung arm. The aficionados are unimpressed, whistling and hooting in derision.

The Doctor's duties and responsibilities for the occasion are clearly diverse, conversations here, consultations there. When the appropriate moment comes he seizes the bridle of the picador's horse and despatches that worthy into the ring with a resounding smack on the flank. The sturdy picador, 'provoker of the bull', jeered and abused throughout the afternoon, does his business as quickly as possible and then withdraws, his face a mask of assumed indifference, as becomes a man accustomed to the total but unmerited disapproval of his fellows.

Suddenly, far left, there is an unscripted commotion as an intruder joins the fray.

'Who is this?' I enquire.

'He is an *espontáneo*,' comes the unsurprised explanation from Aunt Hermenegilda.

And sure enough, the first of many *espontáneos* clambers unsteadily over the barrier into the ring and hurls dust and heavier objects at the departing figure of hate before being bundled out again by the strong arm of the law.

Predictably the pint-sized torero is unable to despatch the valiant *toro* by the sword. After many unsuccessful endeavours he too is joined by several more *espontáneos* eager to voice their opinions and demonstrate their skills, and general confusion ensues. Finally the bull succumbs untidily from its multiple wounds, fatigue, and possibly boredom.

The 'owning syndicate', similarly attired to denote unity, flood into the arena to retake possession of their contribution to the afternoon's entertainment, now inert. Everybody pulls in opposite directions, people fall over in their excitement or for other reasons, photographs are taken and eventually some 450 kilograms of prime steak slide from view.

The afternoon follows its accustomed course. The next torero, from Mexico, despatches his bull with elegant ease, as if to compensate for the first performance. '*¡Aprende!*' shouts my neighbour, 'Learn!'

To the delight of the crowd, one of the fat *banderilleros*, wielders of the mini-spears, gets wedged and stuck behind the safety boards. 'This bullfighter is over weighted,' I am advised by my companions.

Another is insufficiently nimble in the execution of his work and is sent flying by the long sharp horns of one of the bulls. Disconcerted, he staggers away. Nobody helps him.

'Nobody likes him,' explains the Doctor.

Los espontáneos come and go; the bulls come and go. Night falls and the floodlights take over. Alcohol is strictly forbidden in the *plaza*; everybody drinks steadily. It is advisable to leave before the end of proceedings, things have been known to take a turn for the worse. So we slip away, back to the main street in search of a late lunch. Dinner really.

It is cold now, very cold, so La Señora buys scalding *emoliente* and I buy a scarf. The *emoliente* is best described as having the colour of seaweed and the consistency of liquid rubber. My scarf is maroon and I am assured that it is made with the finest alpaca 'from the very young'. Of course. Nobody really knows what *emoliente* is made from, but it is reputedly good for the system.

The Doctor finds soup and trout for us all, then we are ready to go back down the mountain, aided by the light of the half moon and a myriad crystalline stars. La Señora and Aunt Hermenegilda talk on, good shipwreck companions. The Doctor concentrates on lining up for the bridges and negotiating sundry other obstacles.

The return road is long and we are tired. Finally we re-enter Lima to find that surprisingly nothing has changed in the city during our lengthy absence: flashing neon lights and advertising hoardings abound, every second vehicle is a combi belching black fumes. The grimy unwashed buildings, thick with dust, wait on for the balm of rain that will never come.

It is as though we are returning from another world. Which is true. *Me encanta Canta*. We enjoyed our outing to Canta.

But now the Clinic awaits us, scolding our irresponsible absence. The Doctor has been recharged and is ready once again to work his sedate and conscientious way through the lengthy appointment schedules prepared equally conscientiously by Nurse Dulce. Myself, I need to double-check the grease spots in Ernestina's hyperactive ledgers, review the lengthening list of outstanding accounts and then, most importantly, water those vulnerably fragile sweet peas that I planted out last week. As for La Señora, behind closed eyes her mind is quietly ruminating on manifold means whereby she might enhance even further the interior splendour of her palatial enterprise. In the process of such ruminations her thoughts pause coincidentally and not for the first time on the concept of 'the rich man in his castle, the poor man at his gate' and she determines yet again to see to fulfilment her unprecedented vision of funding healthcare centres for the deprived of Peru from the financial success and yet-to-be-realized fortunes of The Ladies' Healthcare Clinic, Lima.

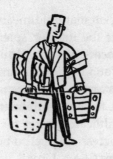

5

Shopping – The Ecstasy

Lima is expanding. Everyone is flocking down from the hills to make their fortune, dreaming that the streets of the city are paved with gold. One day the Limeño tide may turn and everybody will want to move out of town to live up in the hills. But not yet. Why, when Sendero Luminoso, the Shining Path guerrillas, and the equally anarchic movement named after Túpac Amaru, the unsuccessful revolutionary of 1780, are largely defeated terrorist threats of a previous decade, would someone wish to forsake a pastoral life in the majestic mountains of the Andes, abandoning a culture that has withstood the test of centuries, to become an itinerant bubble gum vendor on the streets of Lima? Or to pedal a D'Onofrio ice cream trolley? Or to rummage through the richly stinking garbage bags of San Isidro or Miraflores at dead of night?

'Ah,' I am told, 'you do not understand.' Yes, it is difficult to understand. Is it poverty or immeasurable wealth to lead a life with time to converse, time to think, far removed from sight, smell and sound of traffic, ringed by a far horizon of snow-capped peaks, sharing the moon and the stars at night instead of street lights?

There seem to be almost as many shops and stalls in Lima as there are Limeños. Possibly some people wish there were. La Señora Coraima Pandora del Teodosia Zapallo-Chupado Palermo Bonomini for instance.

'Shopping is my hobby,' she declares in an unguarded moment.

Yes, everybody needs a hobby, like gardening and the bulls and the Doctor. We know that. Then she tries to modify her declaration.

'I am not a high shopper,' she says. 'I am a medium shopper. In fact, I may even call myself a medium-low shopper.'

We listen respectfully. La Señora is an artist. She has never been known to travel in a straight line in thought, word, or deed. And shopping is no exception.

'I only buy what I need,' she states. 'The trouble is, I need everything.' Then, once again she is prompted to amend the text. 'Or rather, our Clinic still needs so many things.' And I think of the fourth-floor store-room, full of discarded computerized bits and bobs, rejected special-effects lights, once-a-year decorations, broken electronic trinkets and the like.

When the shopping mood is on her, La Señora is unstoppable. She simply disappears. For hours. Appointments forgotten, her home, her family, her menagerie of pets and the imported adviser, the Clinic, all abandoned. To cope as best they can. Just as unexpectedly, she reappears.

'Where have you been?' we ask, accusingly.

'Just walking around like an ordinary human being,' she says, lightly.

Not a hint of guilt. She is laden with packages, parcels, boxes and bags. Then she decides to come clean.

'Guess what? Today I went shopping. I went to the Bank, then I turned just a little to the store.'

'How can we pay for all these things?' asks the long-suffering Doctor.

'I cannot be perfect all the time. How can I know?' Always answer a question with a question. La Señora has learnt that domestic trick. She probably invented it. 'I perhaps have many defects,' she says grandly, 'but curiosity is not one of them.' And she knows the script for that exchange as well.

Sometimes the stream of Casa Bonomini guests are the innocent victims of this medium-low shopper.

'La Señora Pelagia Delgado de Yashiyame and La Señora Ximena Guadalupe Peralta de Cuellar came for lunch,' we tell her.

'Oh good,' says La Señora.

'You invited them.'

'Oh. Where are they?' Incuriously incurable.

'They left.'

'Oh.' She has the grace to be momentarily downcast. But only momentarily. 'Come,' she says, brightening. 'See that with these new shoes I am as tall as a tree and I have bought you all a present.'

What can we do? Especially when I discover that I have been presented with a clerical collar, a Bible and a rosary. My grandmother's dream come true.

'You are to wear all these things when you next go out,' I am instructed, before I can draw any other conclusions. 'So that perhaps you will not be attacked and robbed again. And here are some church wafers that I forgot to give you although maybe you don't need them by the moment. I bought them for me but now I lend them to you.'

La Señora prefers to have company on her medium-low shopping safaris. The subliminal principle of collective responsibility, or guilt. And someone to carry the bags. Sometimes it is difficult to refuse. She has tricks and subterfuges.

'I am going shopping,' she announces with an award-winning smile. 'For our Clinic. I think we should buy a new staff intercom system to save running up and down the stairs. And a few flowers and things, of course. Would you like to come?'

'No.' You remember what it was like last time, never mind the intercom. A long-running nightmare. 'I'm too busy. I have to work with Nurse Dulce. I need to analyse her figures.' You have to be cruel to be kind. Anyway, I enjoy analysing Nurse Dulce's figures. Then I remember my manners. 'Thank you for thinking of me. But no. No. No thank you.'

Her face falls. The eyes moisten. You shuffle uncomfortably.

'I see the British winter has crept into your heart,' says La Señora, cast down and avoiding your eye.

You shuffle some more. Then she plays two aces, one after the other.

'They have a sale of training shoes and sports clothes downtown, near that pastry shop, the one with *turrones*, you know, the honey nougat.'

'Well . . . ' Honey nougat! She has caught your interest. New training shoes! Your guard is drooping.

La Señora is one of those people you follow out of curiosity.

'We'll only be half an hour,' she says. 'I go, I look, I come.'

Another ace, a trump too.

'All right then.' Grumpily, beaten by the Roman nuances, the Caesarean echoes. Manners, manners. 'Thank you.' I can look forward to working with Nurse Dulce's figures later.

On occasions the approach is more direct.

'Are you ready?' she demands to know, suddenly appearing at the office door. The advantage of surprise. Maybe La Señora has had secret military training. Possibly as a Special Forces commando. She can probably parachute by night and abseil into occupied territory, or rather, unoccupied defenceless shopping malls. That would explain a lot of things.

'*¿Perdón?* Sorry?' Ambushed. Best to play for time. But the enemy is well trained.

43

'Hurry up! I am rush!'

'But, but . . . ' Floundering. Spluttering. You are doomed. Best to surrender with dignity.

'Now we are leaving. Come!'

'Er, er, where to?' You fire your one last shot. Pathetic. Why not give up like a man?

Either way La Señora is happy. She has someone to carry the bags.

The first deviation from the declared itinerary is not long in coming.

'Señora? Downtown is in the opposite direction.'

She is more than equal to the challenge.

'Please do not speak with me. Today I am in a position of not talking. I am very concentrate. Moreover, I am being pressed by all this traffic.' Then she adds graphically, 'This behind bus is pushing me like a suppository.'

'But . . . '

'When you talk I get distracted, then I don't know where I am coming.'

'What about the car radio? Doesn't that distract you?'

'To the radio I can ignore thinking of the answer so it is not necessary to lower down the volume. With you, you don't let anyone to speak.'

'Oh.'

La Señora is a member of the last-word club.

'Are you here for helping or what? Instead of letting me work, you bother.'

The heaviness of the ensuing silence is the only riposte left open to me. La Señora doesn't even notice, her mind is on the delights that lie ahead.

From time to time La Señora is moved to call on friends in the midst of her shopping marathons. At other times we may happen to find ourselves in a passing museum, although art galleries are the favourite diversion and few are the shopping sorties that are unleavened in this way. With her artistic pedigree La Señora readily instructs me in aspects of the craft that might otherwise have slipped past unnoticed.

'This artist is an abstract,' she explains. 'An abstract is a very deep answer to a proposal. Or perhaps a fake.' Ummm, that rings a bell. 'Of course, some art can be rubbish, but remember that sometimes rubbish can be art.' Ummm again.

Sometimes we are fortunate enough to meet the very artists themselves, to obtain a personal explanation of their pictures. For example:

'This man is my twice-removed cousin,' introduces La Señora. 'He is an artist. You do not know his name.' The introduction has become a non-introduction.

'Hear me this,' says the nameless artistic cousin. 'It was totally amusing to me to paint this work, but of course, humour is a mask for sadness. Today I am with humour. I don't know why, but in this painting here appeared a little fish.' The sadly humorous artist indicates the very spot on the canvas, and then moves on. 'And here is a sort of force,' he reveals, with a sweep of the arm. 'In reality I am not sure where it came from or indeed where it is going. And this here is a rat, it is sign-bolic. Now I must go, excuse me so much. My wife is requiring for me. In life everything has to end.'

Sometimes the diversions are prompted by other forces.

'In this hour I must eat something,' declares La Señora. It is not an unknown occurrence. 'Except these roads are not my territory, I do not know their movements. Please hold on to your everythings or you may lose them over these bumps. And this traffic is so aggressive, maybe they are waiting to go home. We are driving fine here, it is the others all around. See this combi is coming to the road without putting the blinking marker. He obligates me to move. But in these circumstances Dr Hermogenes says "Don't horn, don't horn!" But I cannot be silent in this situation. This is too much for me, so I horn.' And she does.

Sometimes we lose our way.

'I am sorry for this big ride but I got lost,' says our leader. 'Now we stop a little and we may seek assistance.' And so saying she winds down the car window. 'To reach the Santa Rosa restaurant,' she enquires of a passer-by, 'how to go?'

'Oh, you just follow the road,' answers the passer-by helpfully.

'I need Avenida Santander.'

'This is Avenida Santa Cruz.'

'Yes, I know, but I need Santander.'

'No, this is Santa Cruz.'

'Thank you.'

'No need to thank, it was a pleasure.'

La Señora winds up the window. 'That conversation,' she explains, 'it didn't conclude.'

It was a Peruvian conversation.

The excursion unfolds, and unfolds. To discourage the possibility of further questioning La Señora resorts to any flight of fancy that happens to cross her mind.

'Here in Peru we are not allowed to talk in the car. If the Polices see too much talking they may stop us. There! Feel what a marvellous quietness.'

Once parked, my job is to trot behind with the packages, but occasionally I am favoured with a word or two of encouragement, explanation or exhortation.

Such as: 'The pastry shop should still be open when we arrive.'

Or: 'These bargains are very cheap money.'

Or: 'Do not press me on the hour, Mr British. Don't press me for time, don't be a timed person, do not mark your life with a watch like a watch watcher. The time you never did allow me. Wait please and let me plan the future. Just now we are in a terrible moment. We are shopping for a wedding present and I am very hurried and approaching a breakdown nervous. And now on top of everything I feel I am going to sneeze my nose. Oh! I hate sneezing. I really don't have the time to sneeze.'

All this just in case it might cross my mind to show any sign of impatience.

Whenever possible, La Señora likes to bargain, even without any intention of buying.

'I see here your house is for sale,' she says, for example, addressing a new-found street acquaintance, adding mendaciously, 'I am for you a probable buyer.' Then she explains her technique. 'I make a small offering, they answer me upset, I answer them upset, again they answer me upset. This is the trick. Then I say nothing and they say nothing. Just "thank you". Remember this.'

I will.

The medium-low shopper is not only active in Lima. For her it is a global hobby; for others it is a matter of global concern. It's just a question of perspective. The Doctor apparently spent his honeymoon personally carrying two enormous cast-iron storks across Europe. That was three decades ago and now the storks are standing in the entrance hall of Casa Bonomini, going visibly rusty in the humidity that is Lima, but for the Doctor the invisible mental scars are incalculable, with or without humidity.

'Yes,' confirms La Señora brightly, 'those storks they remind him of our honeymoon.'

It's true. When pressed he can relate the tale as vividly as though it happened yesterday.

Nothing surprises him any more. On a recent trip to trace her family roots and gaze upon the ancestral castle in Sweden, La Señora left with one suitcase and returned with five. Nothing surprises the Doctor any more.

'Each time I come from the travels,' says La Señora, almost defensively but not quite, 'I bring the things which are very happy to be sitting in my house. It is not a punishment to travel and carry.'

The Doctor looks thoughtful.

On a loosely styled business trip to Tumbes, on the coast in the far north of Peru, we pause from extolling the exceptional virtues of the Clinic by means of selectively distributing our newly and proudly produced promotional brochure to prospective clients to buy waves of discontented lobsters and great scurries of bad-tempered crabs, boxes and boxes of seafood to be transported back to Lima. The bargains are declared to be irresistible (in this comparable to the blandishments contained in the ten-page glossy brochure – including as it does surgical illustrations that appear to have been culled from the internet and possibly even borrowed from rival publications, as well as appealing photographs of the Doctor and the English consultant gazing out from across their empty desks with suitable gravitas).

'You just can't imagine how delicious these are,' says La Señora. 'Of course, I am allergic to lobsters, but what can I do?'

Obviously there are allergies and allergies. Incidentally but equally inconveniently we also acquire two dozen large coconut palms for a minor horticultural enterprise La Señora has conceived. Perhaps there are plans for a coconut stall in the Clinic. Who knows? Maybe Fidel will plant them, maybe they will die.

We arrive at the airport for the homeward flight, accompanied by what must have been at least a football team of seafood and coconut palm porters. La Señora sails ahead; she needs to make a few last-minute purchases in the terminal shops.

I call after her plaintively. 'What shall I do with all these men?'

'Pay them!' comes the imperious response.

Stupid question, I suppose. I pay them, pathetic to the last.

Travelling through Chiclayo, again in northern Peru, again on promotional business passing round the smart brochures to friends of friends and to La Señora's seemingly endlessly extending extended family, I am once more the duty donkey.

As it happens, Chiclayo is good for rice. It grows well there. It's the climate. On a purely personal basis I am sorry for this.

After careful research La Señora buys two enormous sacks of the finest quality grain. I am not sure if they are avoirdupois or metric, but it matters not. They are hugely heavy.

Our next stop is Trujillo, 200 kilometres south down *la costa*. We take a motor taxi to the bus station. The rice has pride of place in the three-wheeled conveyance, the gallant *chofer* surely suffers a slipped disc or a hernia, or both, and we nearly have to walk behind. *Tourismo del Norte* is the grandiose claim that I read on the back of the motorized tricycle, but I am not in the mood to be impressed.

'This rice is of the finest quality,' says La Señora, in case I had missed the point. 'You just cannot believe how good it is.'

Not without difficulty the straining bus driver loads the two sacks into his baggage compartment as the *chofer* hobbles back to his motor taxi. We are in process of leaving a trail of disgruntled cripples in our wake.

It is the same story in Trujillo: bus, motor taxi, hotel. In the best spirit of Peruvian hospitality everyone is anxious to assist the gringo, until they feel the weight of the sacks. The equally heavy expense in tips is mounting rapidly, even in advance of compensation claims for bodily injury and the purchase of comforting trusses. La Señora finally surrenders.

'This fine rice we should send by bus to Lima in advance of our leaving. It will travel overnight and be there before us.'

Or even in advance of our coming. Thankfully I bid farewell to the two unrepentant fat sacks, which are becoming heavier by the minute. In Lima, the Doctor impassively collects the fine rice in the big, once-white truck, by which time it has become the most expensive grain in the city. But La Señora is at least right on one count. It is delicious.

Admittedly the principal beneficiary of La Señora's shopping largesse is indeed normally our Clinic, healthcare showcase of the imminent future and intended centre of unimagined excellence. Day by day it becomes ever more lavish, true to our concept of providing a home-from-home for the well-heeled ladies, where we constantly endeavour to surprise our patients by treating them as individuals. However, whether we really need quite such a profusion of flowing floral arrangements, decorative statues, grand ornaments and other objets d'art to achieve this illusion is perhaps debatable. Nonetheless, and indisputably, our reputation blossoms and the metaphorical turnstiles tick merrily, as well they need to in view of our perilous banking predicament. We have opened and we are running, and I scarcely notice that the six-month point of my six-week assignment has been and gone. Whether I am one of the staff or one of the pets matters not. I feel in no hurry to be gone. Maybe I should have brought that second suitcase after all.

Occupied with his patients, the expectant, wishful and wistful, the ever-popular Doctor is very much in the forefront of this burgeoning activity. But like a long-distance runner he paces himself well and notwithstanding his crowded appointment book his closed-door consultations are long and unhurried. In rare moments of repose he has the illusive trick, probably perfected when he was excelling at medical school, of sitting in his consulting chair holding a reference book or professional journal and sleeping soundly.

'Dr Hermogenes,' I ask, knocking and entering, 'am I disturbing you?' His eyelids flicker and he shakes his head. 'You were reading with your eyes shut.'

'No, no,' he says, calmly corrective, but nonetheless inadvertently turning a page backwards. However, he makes a quick recovery. 'When I study,' he hastens to explain, 'I come from the back to the front.'

Whilst pondering the obstetrical relevance of this, I chance to discover that one of the secrets of the Doctor's enduring stamina is his double life.

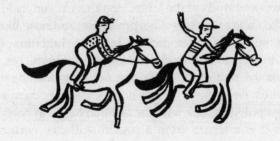

6

El Hipódromo de Monterrico

For La Señora, the Clinic is a dream come true. Since those years long ago when she accompanied Dr Hermogenes to the United States to ease him through to success in the completion of his higher medical studies she had cherished the vision of presenting him with a Clinic truly befitting his talents. She was also possessed of her wider philanthropic dream: that of devoting the profits from the enterprise to found and fund primary healthcare centres dedicated to the poor and needy. Thus impelled, hers became the creative force that for more than a decade had surmounted all obstacles to build the Ladies' Healthcare Clinic, Lima, hers was the hand that held the pen that sketched the graceful lines of the edifice and ordered the juxtapositioning of the component parts, visions that were subsequently passed to a ghost architect to translate into hard-lined building plans and concrete via drawing board, T-square and rule. And now, at long last, here she is, but a hop and a skip and a bank loan away from her goal.

Dr Hermogenes also has his dreams. Those arduous years of

hard work and study at the Johns Hopkins University Hospital have taken him to the top of his profession and now, like many another successful man before him, he harbours restless desires to be something else, someone different. Yes, in his case, it is the pull of the bulls. But not only does he want to breed bulls, he hankers to rear horses. Perhaps there is some deep psychological link with the fact that he is a gynaecologist. Perhaps it is a legacy from a previous life, or perhaps it is a wish to be fulfilled in some future existence. However, as things stand, he is a physician of note and the extension of this activity to embrace bulls and horses is not without its difficulties.

Some might say that gynaecology, horses and bulls make strange bedfellows, although from the depth of his long experience the Doctor would opine that this is not necessarily so and he is undaunted. In silent pursuit of his aspirations he favours the big, once-white truck as a mode of transport in preference to arriving at the Clinic in a sedate saloon. Pictures and paintings of rampant bulls and thrusting matadors find their way into his consulting room. Every morning on rising he is inclined to select cord trousers and a tasselled leather belt from his wardrobe instead of a suit and tie.

None of which meets with the unqualified approval of La Señora. It is difficult for her to do anything about the big, once-white truck, but she mounts periodic frontal assaults on the choice of belt and cord trousers, and launches lightning cloak-and-dagger swoops against the pictures, which she confiscates on the grounds that they are 'inappropriate'. Whereupon the Doctor adopts a heavily depressed countenance as he goes glumly about his duties, hemmed in by the cheerless and aggressively stripped walls of his workplace, constantly reminded that nudity is like a good chocolate pudding – totally captivating but best in small helpings. The situation is invariably saved after a few days when the soft-hearted

Señora is beset by remorse at the suffering she is causing and returns the offending articles, which in any case have become a thoroughgoing nuisance littering the floor and cluttering the corners of her office where they have been ineffectively hidden.

The Doctor's farm is a more intractable hurdle. It is not insubstantial in size, although to the untutored eye it is a desert really, making the precise dimensions of limited academic relevance. Nevertheless, there it lies, about 100 kilometres down the coastal road to the south of Lima, and Dr Hermogenes is at peace on the arid acres. Given the opportunity he will disappear before dawn on Sundays, not reappearing in the city until after dark, tired and dusty but happy of heart. What he does all day when he is at the farm, or in the desert, nobody knows. No consulting rooms, no prolonged personal appointments; just the farm men to talk to and, as the Doctor is pleased to explain, lots of things to be done, generally speaking. Veritably a thousand things without a name. Certainly the big, once-white truck always bears evidence of much activity, laden with sacks of feed on the outward journey, littered with straw and hay on the return.

Then there are the filthy pigs that live on the farm. Sometimes the Doctor brings one of them back to the house, like an unexpected and unwilling guest.

'This a pork to eat,' he announces proudly. And we do. 'At London, you call them pigs or porks?' he wonders, apropos of nothing.

'It all depends on context,' I tell him helpfully and Dr Hermogenes nods thoughtfully, filing away the information in his encyclopaedic mind.

The Doctor is known in all the villages that surround the farm. From time to time he is presented with small tokens of great esteem, such as choice cuts of meat, bulging bags of overweight vegetables and other abundant produce, in anticipation of possible reciprocal favours in the future. It is the way.

'Today they gave me cheese and a turkey. It is alive, but it is a turkey. And the cheese is hard cheese from the goat. I tell you that in case you think it is soft cheese.'

'And the turkey, can we eat it?'

'One day we can. But first it needs to be increased. I put it on the farm.'

At present there are no bulls on the farm but horses there are. Several, swishing their languid tails against the irritable flies, moving from side to side of the paddock on irregular impulse with a double dip of the head.

The Doctor is in league with a mysterious Chinaman, code name Mickey Moto. Mr Moto sells sanitary ware: pipes, basins, lavatory pans and other handy items and he too hankers after an alternative life. Understandably. In his case, he dreams of being a racehorse owner, although in this instance the subliminal psychological link with lavatory pans in particular and his profession in general is not so readily apparent. It is of no importance. The symbiotic agreement means that the horses are produced from somewhere by Mickey Moto and the Doctor keeps them on the farm until the moment is right. Then, whenever that may be, they go back to the Chinaman for intensive training and finally they are raced in Lima at the Hipódromo de Monterrico. Whereupon, the prize money is shared and the process repeated. Simple.

Putting it mildly, or even less than mildly, which is more often the case, La Señora has reservations about the scheme. She has even more reservations about Mrs Mickey Moto, who has good legs and wears short skirts.

Nonetheless, the Doctor and Mr Moto work industriously on their plan. The Doctor, as ever, rises early, the horses are carefully prepared and rehearsed (with Dr Desastre being co-opted as ex-officio dietary consultant), and the weeks pass with mounting anticipation.

Serendipitously, our patients at the Clinic are notoriously bad timekeepers (matched only by the dilatory settlement of their accounts), a not entirely uncommon manifestation in private healthcare; but far from being an inconvenience the resultant gaps that appear in the appointments schedule are welcomed by Dr Hermogenes and put to good effect. He seizes these opportunities to slip out unannounced, supposedly on urgent clinical errands but in fact to oversee the affairs of the syndicate, double-checking on vital equine matters, such as the provision of fortified oats, no doubt, and probably administering last-minute booster shots of high octane, whilst it falls to doe-eyed Nurse Dulce to maintain sweet-natured calm in the now rapidly filling Reception.

When all is ready for the first event, eager Dr Vonday is left in charge of the empty Clinic and we head for the racecourse. La Señora is not in the best of humours, the Doctor has difficulty suppressing his excitement, and I am unrealistically hopeful, as always.

El Hipódromo de Monterrico is truly a racecourse on a grand scale. Vast echoing stands with an enormously optimistic capacity for thousands of equally optimistic punters, beautiful grounds, lovely trees and gardens, completely irrelevant.

'About 1967,' the Doctor tells me from memory, 'that's when it was built. It was the biggest in all South America. In those days we had no games in Lima, no casinos. Here was very full. You needed to wear a top and a tie. There was nice catering. Nowadays everything is decreased, standards have fallen.'

True, I thought, glancing round, nowadays everywhere you look it is decreased. As with our Clinic, the national economy, or rather, the absence of, is threatening to take its toll like a baleful hurricane lurking to seaward. Nevertheless, La Señora, with half an eye on the possibility of photographic coverage and even of television interviews, has dressed appropriately for the occasion.

'With this parasol I feel like an antique lady,' she observes, the mauve and violet cherries on her enormous straw-brimmed sunhat nodding in obeisance.

We promptly demur, of course, ignoring the enveloping presence of the Lima mist, *la neblina*, rolling resolutely down the racecourse and totally obscuring the remotest possibility of any sunshine, if not for a month, certainly for the day.

We meet up with Mickey Moto. Mrs Moto is also there, looking very charming in, yes, a short skirt. Our horse is called Rescate. 'Rescue', or more precisely, 'Ransom'. Very apt. We need the money. We go down to the paddock. Rescate looks nervous. We meet the trainer. Now I am nervous. He has one of those weathered South American faces made from well-preserved leather. Give him a few more years and he will look like a peripatetic raisin. I notice that he doesn't look us in the eye. We all expect nothing. But of course, we have our dreams. And I look at the winner's enclosure and I dream some more.

Well, Rescate does his best. There are a dozen runners and he is last. By quite a long way. But he does his best.

Two months later we are back at El Hipódromo. Dr Vonday is back at base; he likes race days. We are all dreaming again. This time it is just me and the Doctor. And our new horse, optimistically, or perhaps euphemistically, named Expectativa. No Mr and Mrs Moto. They have gone mysteriously to Miami. No La Señora. She was disappointed with us last time. Nothing mysterious about that. The parasol has been returned to the loft.

'This Classic Race is just for women,' explains the Doctor, 'and this little horse comes well at the end.'

I look at him quizzically.

'She comes good from behind,' adds the Doctor, in amplification. 'But note that this horse is a very small size.'

We go down to the paddock. The Doctor rehearses the race strategy with the jockey.

'Stay in the back until the Coca-Cola sign.'

The jockey nods and leaps up on to Expectativa.

'Very elastic man, heh?' observes the Doctor.

It's true, very elastic. We meet another owner. He is number 6, we are number 1.

'Suerte, Doctor.'

'Gracias, señor. Tu tambien.'

'Good luck, Doctor.' 'Thank you. You too.' Of course, but not too much. The eyes do not meet. We expect nothing; dreaming is free.

The strategy goes nicely until we get to the Coca-Cola sign. Expectativa is definitely at the back. But there she stays, all the way to the tape. Well, she picks up a couple of places, but it is not enough.

Driving home in the big, once-white truck we talk of other things. I resist the temptation to suggest to the Doctor that we might get some bulls for the farm. And as for cautions about fast women and slow horses, it's not the time for repeating that cliché either. We come to a tacit understanding to dream on.

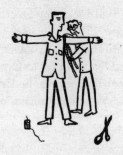

7

Shopping – The Agony

Addict or otherwise, for every shopper the moment arrives when the choice has been made and there is a need to pay up and go, like leaving a restaurant after an enjoyable meal. But in Peru the process is not that simple.

'*¿Efectivo o tarjeta?*' asks the cashier. Cash or card?

'Whatever.'

'*¿Boleto o factura?*'

'I'm sorry?'

'*¿Boleto o factura?*' It's a device for reclaiming sales tax rather than an invitation to dance.

'OK, *factura.*' Whatever, again.

'*Uh huh. ¿Razón Social y RUC, por favor?*'

'I JUST WANT TO PAY THE BILL! ' You regret your impatience immediately. Everybody in the store looks at you. There is an uncomfortable silence.

'I'm sorry, I didn't mean to shout. But I want to pay and go home. I only bought three crayons.'

The tension eases. Just a touch. But rules are rules. In case of interruption, return to the top of the page.

'*¿Efectivo o tarjeta?*' enquires the cashier. Cash or card?

There is no escape. Learn the catechism or you won't get your crayons. No colouring for you today.

That's the easy part. Try visiting *la ferretería*, the ironmonger.

Check La Señora's list. Some of these screws, some of those, some of those nails, some of these. And while you're there, some of this and some of that, plus a few metres of the green cable for the new big screen in the auditorium that will relay surgical secrets from the operating theatre to invited medical audiences and that will also prove a real boon for World Cup matches, and some of the red, and better take some of the other, just in case. And oh yes, and oh yes! There, nothing else, that's it, perfect. You are ready with the catechism, ready with the cash.

Not so fast, señor! The sales clerk looks suspiciously at your varied selection and reaches for the biro. Ah, the store man has just borrowed it for a moment, *un ratito*. Of course, *un ratito*, one moment. There we are, there's the sleepy store man, here's the unbelievable one and only biro. Now, let's see . . . the mobile phone rings, the cellular.

In Peru, when the cellular calls, the world stops. It's a cultural thing, you see. More recent than the Incas but as deeply ingrained as a Cusco carving. Not so very long ago the waiting time for obtaining a telephone line in Lima was a couple of years, or more. That's if you happened to have the money to hand, the readies ready, about 3,000 US dollars. Then came the advent of the glorious cellular and the rest is history. The great communications love affair. True, it's universal, but Peruvians are particularly passionate about it. Who could be that much in love with a cellular? Well, come to Lima and find out. They take them everywhere, to the gym, to the dinner table, to the cinema, to the beach. You even receive calls from people sitting in the dentist's chair (e.g. La Señora), and yes, definitely from friends sitting in the bathroom. That's another global perversion. Drowned mobiles are commonplace. They have even been found discarded in lavatory cisterns, innocent victims of heaven knows what domestic discords. And of course Peruvians go to bed with their mobile phones. Constantly. Why not? You can do a lot worse than that. At least they don't snore. Some people sleep with teddy bears.

Needless to say, La Señora is the proud possessor of a fistful of cellulars. They come and they go: lost, abandoned, forgotten, reappearing and rediscovered. But regardless of what mode they are in, not for one moment do they cease the demands of their inanely insistent ringing, usually at the most inopportune of moments. This is how it goes.

'I have wonderful news for you,' declares La Señora breathlessly, exploding into the room.

'Tell me,' I respond, calm and cool as a stereotype but prepared to be quite interested and laying down my quill.

'I believe this news will change your life.'

'Really? Tell me all.' Now I too am breathless. Almost.

'Right! Listen carefully, and make a note of the figures.'

As bidden, I re-reach for the quill. At that moment one of the cellulars springs to life and La Señora is compelled to answer. Twenty minutes later the animated exchange is completed.

'That was the Bank,' explains La Señora. 'They didn't say anything really. Just talking.'

I knew it. 'Good,' I reply from the edge of my chair, in no way dismissive and without a hint of impatience. 'But what about this other news?'

'What other news? Please do not delay me in this moment, I have many shoppings to attend to, or rather, to which I must attend.'

For some time I have been the only person in all Peru without a cellular. Like the Queen in England, I imagine. Then, for reasons best forgotten, I decide to advance myself. I visit Telefónica, money changes hands and I wait for my life to change. Nothing happens. This clever little telephone will ring for you all over South America, that's what they told me. Quite aside from the marked lack of interest and demand I soon discover that the clever little gadget refuses to function outside Lima. So I return to the sales office to adjust the programming. That has to be the answer. The programming.

'Your telephone is fine,' the company girl tells me.

'Oh good,' I say, 'except that it doesn't work.'

'Well, then you should go back to the jungle and try again.'

'But I have done that twice and I am politely telling you it doesn't work,' say I, ignoring the inference of the jungle jibe.

'Your telephone is fine.'

'May I have my money back, then? In return you may have your telephone back. It's fine.'

'Certainly not. And please be careful with your words which are bordering on the disrespectful.'

'Inviting me to go back to the jungle is not a solution to the problem.'

'When you are there, if your telephone still has a difficulty then you may ring this special number.'

'Thank you. Why don't we ring it now?'

'You have to be in the jungle to prove that your telephone, which is fine, doesn't work.'

'But how can I ring that number if my telephone isn't working? Would it be too disrespectful if I ask to speak to the supervisor?'

'No.'

'No I can't or no it wouldn't?'

'Next please.'

Back to the jungle. I knew it was folly to have bought a cellular; now I must suffer the rightful nemesis for harbouring desires above my station.

Going about your business in Peru there are rare moments when you get a fleeting suspicion that perhaps in some quarters customer satisfaction is not the highest of priorities. On the occasion that I need a domicile certificate from the local police station I am directed to make payment for this insignificant service at the nearby Banco de la Nación. I walk the five blocks as directed and on arrival find a dense line of people circling the outside of the bank, like film extras auditioning for a re-enactment of Custer's Last Stand, or as though tickets for a pop concert or a football match had just gone on sale. Yes, I am assured, this is the queue to get inside. So I add my presence to the motley throng and wait, shuffling forward at intervals. Customers or cattle? Either way, it's milking time. Finally it is my turn to be admitted to the inner portals, only to find another long line snaking round the interior of the bank. There are just three cashiers in attendance to serve the several hundred waiting postulants. Nobody complains; it's the way things are, so why complain? On the wall to the side of the endless queue is a box ironically marked 'Suggestions'. No one is inclined to waste more time by using it; no point in stating the obvious to deaf ears. The cost of my form is the price of half a saucer of coffee; the cost in time is less than half a day, but not by much.

Anyway, back here in *la ferretería* our sales clerk is on his cellular (which is clearly fine) and his world has stopped. Ours too, incidentally. Apparently, the words: 'I'm busy right now, can you ring me back?' do not exist in Castellano. There is no known translation. Unfortunately. Maybe there is a presidential decree forbidding Peruvians from turning off their cellulars. Maybe the mobile phones in Peru are made without an 'off' switch. Who knows? Except that you are waiting for the sales clerk, who is on his cellular.

Eventually the call ends (probably the battery ran out), and the writing starts. By hand, with the shop biro, now returned by the dozy store man. Everything is itemized. You regret your capricious choices of a little of this and a little of that. But you have learnt not to shout. It doesn't help, it confuses. Just rehearse your shopping mantra, 'Everything is temporary', over and over again. That helps. And remember to bring a good book with you next time. That would also help.

To lighten the mood and for a little diversion, try visiting El Mundo Cosmético in Avenida Petit Thouars. There is no escaping the *boleto/factura* routine but here the real entertainment starts when you attempt to pay the bill.

You are waved towards a large mirror at the end of the shop in which someone has carefully cut a mousehole-sized aperture at waist level. Through this, into the darkness beyond, you push your *boleto/factura* which is suddenly invisibly snatched from your grasp, only to reappear with a disembodied index finger tapping the total due. While you gaze in startled amazement, the tapping index finger is joined by a thumb which rubs to and fro, so you respond to the international language and pass the appropriate money into the mousehole. There is a pause, then, everything checked and in order, out comes the index finger again, motioning you to the side to collect your purchases. You get the message and move as indicated, only to be rewarded by an encouraging thumbs-up from the mousehole. Somewhat mesmerized, you gather your bag of goodies and head for home, chancing a backward glance at the mouse house. A triumphant Churchillian V-sign pops out of the void to send you on your way rejoicing.

At the door of the shop you essay another sidelong glance in the direction of the magical mirror. But that's it. Nothing stirs in the darkness of the cavity. Game over. Maybe you imagined the whole performance.

After all those adventures, you should be thankful you are not in the pharmacy. Why? Well, just imagine that you are, for example, in Mr Wong's nice pharmacy. You need a caress or two of mollifying balm for some anxious haemorrhoids. For your friend's restless haemorrhoids, that is. There is just one pharmacist on duty so you loiter, waiting for a more intimate moment. But the pharmacy is busy, the intimate moment never comes. So you have to take your place in the line. When your turn comes, you state your business, confidentially.

'*¿Qué?*' asks the pharmacist loudly. '*¿Hemorroides?*'

'Yes, for my friend.'

'*¡Ah, almorranas!*'

'*Sí*, piles, for my friend.'

Off he goes and you feel the pharmacy group eyeing you doubtfully. Don't they know that half the people in this world have piles and that the other half are liars?

Back comes the pharmacist with a well-marked tube of the required palliative. You reach out, gratefully. Wrong. First the paperwork, then to another line to pay the pretty cashier. She reads your *boleto* (or is it a *factura*?) with distaste and avoids your eye. You want to explain about your friend, but she doesn't give you the opportunity. You are condemned. Anyway, back to the pharmacist, all done at last. Wait your turn. The pharmacist remembers you.

'*¡Ah, almorranas!*' he declares in that quite unnecessarily loud voice of his, as though it is your name, Señor Almorranas, picking up the big, well-marked soothing tube and waving it into a plastic bag. Transparent, of course. It doesn't matter any more. The whole of Lima knows about your friend's irritating condition. Mr Piles, are you sitting comfortably?

There's just one thing more. You have forgotten that your money is in your sock. Remember? Yes, you don't like money belts, which proclaim to the world: 'I am a tourist and here are my valuables.' And anyway, they make you look pregnant. Ever since you were robbed at Morro Solar you have kept your money in your sock, with just 10 nuevos soles in your pocket ready for the next mugger, to avoid any unpleasantness. The trouble is, the money has a habit of going further and further down into your shoe when you walk, just like one of those ears of barley, in reverse, that used to go up your sleeve like a caterpillar on school walks in the country half a century ago. There's nothing else for it, you have to take your shoe off to pay the bill. The eyes of the pharmacy group open wide in amazement. These gringos with *almorranas*, how they suffer!

Even that's not the end of it. As is the custom in Peru, the cashier holds your proffered note up to the light to see if it is a forgery. It's just the way things are, call it tradition if you like, there's no need to take it personally. But of course you do. The cheek of it!

Then the cashier checks the quality of the paper, frowns and passes the note questioningly to the big-hipped supervisor. The pantomime is re-enacted. The pharmacy group are riveted, expectant, hopeful for further embarrassment. But the matronly supervisor disappoints them and gives the note the green light.

'*Húmedo*,' she pronounces with a dismissive toss, haughty horse that she is. Just a little humid. And probably a bit niffy to boot. Well, what do they expect? It's not your fault, it's been in your shoe, hasn't it?

You take your change with a flouncy flick in return and hold the notes up to the light to check for forgeries. But the interest has gone, nobody cares and it doesn't have the same effect. Do what you like. And by the way, señor, is this transparent bag containing this unpleasant-looking tube of haemorrhoid balm yours by any chance? Yes! No! It's for my friend, you see, he's the one with the piles! But the pretty assistant isn't listening. Oh! The utter shame of it all.

By the very nature of things, there have to be happier days. Like when the zip maestro mends my favourite long-serving

65

zipper bag. Joy. That bag had been half-broken for years and I had despaired in at least half a dozen countries of ever getting it repaired. A real wizard is the zip maestro. An unacclaimed Peruvian national treasure.

Then comes the instance of my favourite long-serving desert boots. Encouraged by the zip experience, I take them to the *zapatero*.

'These boots, they squeeze too much? *¿Sí o no?*' enquires the shoemaker.

'No,' I tell him, 'they need to be resoled.'

'*¡Ah! Sí,*' says *el zapatero,* '*por supuesto.*' Of course. He reaches into the convenient cupboard behind him and without even turning to look, his hand triumphantly finds just what is required, two matching soles. Tomorrow? Marvellous. We agree the price and the hour. Marvellous again.

'*Hasta mañana.*'

'*Sí, hasta mañana.*' Until tomorrow.

On the morrow, I return. There are the pieces of my boots; there is the *zapatero*. But where are the soles? The shoemaker looks at me.

'These,' he says accusingly, indicating the boots, 'are Size 9.' I nod in agreement. Same as my feet. 'And these,' he says protectively, producing and waving his pair of matching soles, 'are Size 8.'

Impasse. I gather up the pieces of my favourite desert boots. One of life's little disappointments. And a right little disaster is the boot maestro.

It is almost the same story with my new shirt. I take the material to *el sastre* in Miraflores; the tailor makes the shirt. Hand-made, a fraction of the price of Jermyn Street. As it happens, on this occasion the cuffs are a mite tight, hand-made for Matchstick Man. Leave it to me, indicates *el sastre*. Fix it in a jiffy. *¿Un ratito? ¡Exacto!* Tomorrow? *¡Sí, mañana! ¡Perfecto!* Not only a new shirt, but also my Español is coming along nicely.

On the morrow, I return. There is my nice blue shirt on its hanger; there is *el sastre*. The only thing that catches my eye is that my nice blue shirt, hand-made, now has short sleeves, summer barbecue-style. *El sastre* certainly doesn't catch my eye. He looks down and fiddles with his tape measure. Finally he speaks.

'Do you have any more of that blue material?' he enquires nervously, still measuring imaginary waists, chests and inside legs.

'NO! ¡NO!' I do not repeat myself. I say it twice for the sake of emphasis, once in English, once in Spanish. Bilingual to highlight the point.

El sastre stops fiddling abruptly. He is unaccustomed to violence in his *sastrería*.

'¿No?' he whispers, eyes wide. '¡No!' He repeats himself, in Spanish. And probably wets himself, inadvertently.

'NO!' Then I translate, more quietly but with equal menace. '*No.*' I cleverly sense that the conversation is going nowhere.

Now I have a new tailor, Isaac, and a new short-sleeved blue shirt for summer barbecues. I share Isaac with the Doctor and we are having new suits made. The Doctor has gone for a sort of green, which surprises me; I have ended up with a sort of brown, which surprises him. Isaac takes everything in his stride, and commends us both on the excellence of the cloth and on our subtle choice of colours. He is a traditional bespoke tailor of the old school. Just a little overweight.

'Sometimes with the belly pushing through the shirt,' observes the Doctor, with the uncomfortable clinical exactitude of his profession.

Isaac does house calls, as doctors used to do in olden times, generally arranging his schedule around his siesta and avoiding the heat of the day. Mouth full of pins, well over 100 years old, he puffs his way up to the top floor of the Clinic, my office doubling as the fitting and cutting room on these occasions, coincidental and totally unconnected with the precedent established in the former Savile Row map room of the Royal Geographical Society.

'His cheeks are heavy,' explains La Señora, observing Isaac's arrival. 'He cannot talk.'

In the tranquil ambience of the fourth floor the suits are making good progress. The Doctor, more or less safe from prowling patients at this altitude, is in philosophical mood for his fitting. 'I have suits from when I was single, but I cannot get in. I have the pants from my wedding, but also I cannot get in.'

Isaac is pleased with the work-in-progress. '¡*Perfecto!*' he breathes, from every standpoint.

With a keen eye La Señora points out all the defects, and now there are many, and Isaac is less pleased. But his mouth is full of pins and he is disadvantaged. He is further disadvantaged when he is supposedly struck down with a hernia. On receipt of the news we sympathize, but the fact remains that the green and brown production line has come to an unscheduled halt. It was bound to happen, I suppose. Fate has decreed that the half-finished sort-of-green and sort-of-brown suits should never see the light of day, never walk the pavements of Lima. Yet another of life's little disappointments. On second thoughts, perhaps it was La Señora rather than Fate who sounded the death knell for the suits, a secret veto on account of colour and general unsuitability.

Christmas will soon be on us, but I may give shopping a miss this year. More immediately, the Lima bullfighting season is already upon us, the zenith of the Doctor's calendar and rich source of sustenance to his alter ego. As is becoming our habit, we need no second bidding to escape from the demands of the

Clinic, more time-consuming than onerous. Not because we feel that the success of the enterprise is assured, rather in response to a collective urge to flee the realities of stressful spreadsheets that are anything but balanced and cash flow projections that reveal a minimum of flow and even less cash.

Accordingly, all appointments are rescheduled, Dr Vonday, ever the bridesmaid, is deputed to take the non-existent strain and we head for the exit, extending deaf ears to the disapproving tut-tutting of Señorita Hilda, inseparably laden with all manner of documents of the utmost import, as she watches our waywardly light-hearted departure.

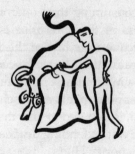

8

La Feria del Señor de los Milagros

The Lima bullfighting season is short: just six weekends in October and November. *Las corridas de toros* take place in the city's historic Plaza de Acho, well over 200 years old, the mecca of Peruvian bullfighting. It is the oldest bullring in the Americas, dating from 1766, the zenith of Spanish colonization in Peru. Carlos III on the throne of Spain, George III on the throne of England. The American War of Independence looming to the north.

Dr Hermogenes is not only an aficionado of the sport, he is a *conocedor*, one who knows. Bullfighting is about knowing and understanding. Ask any matador, ask the Doctor, and they will talk late into the night. There is a mystique to bullfighting, dark elements, primitive forces of life and death.

The Doctor buys our tickets early and never misses a *corrida*. The tickets are marked *Sol*, *Sombra*, and *Sol y Sombra*. You can sit in the sun, in the shade, or in a little of each as the sun marks the course of the afternoon. On cool days the *Sol* is nice, on hot days a little of the *Sombra* is more comfortable. The Doctor invariably opts for the shade, right at the top of the steeply banked seats. He finds that advice and suggestions travel better on a downward trajectory. Furthermore, anyone unwise enough to engage him in verbal fisticuffs is seriously disadvantaged as they twist uncomfortably in their place, craning upwards, competing against gravity as well as reason.

Moreover, from that elevated vantage point La Señora can communicate more easily with her many friends. Including the *ambulantes*, the vendors of drinks, chocolate and ices who skip nimbly up and down the tiered rows. They all know her, the harvest of years of faithful attendance.

'¡*Oye, Gordita!*' she calls. Hey, Little Fattie! Or even more complimentary, '¡*Oye, Gorda linda!*' Hey, beautiful Fattie! '¡*Oye, Sambo!*'

Peruvians feel no obligation to complicate their lives with the fetters of political correctness. All the necessities of existence are cheerfully delivered and everyone is happy, especially the Doctor with his habitual and enormous postprandial cigar.

An essential prelude to *las corridas* is a good lunch, which ensures that everyone arrives in fine form. So we have our good lunch, at the Mesón Los Angeles (Proprietress: the melodic Miriam Portocarrero Llontop – a name to conjure with), and then we struggle belatedly in the stream of vehicles crossing the Rimac river. Rafael the driver is reassuring that we will arrive in time, if not on time.

'I am like Niggle Mansell. This bus here, he is also going to the bulls.'

En route we encounter an unwelcome slice of Lima life. Stationary at the lights, an *ambulante* passes a flyer through the

71

driver's open window. Just another leaflet for a pizza house or something. We receive it courteously. Everybody needs to earn their *cebiche*. At that moment, unexpectedly, another *ambulante* bangs loudly on the offside roof of the car. We all turn. Except for streetwise Medical Student One. He is alert to the trick and calls a warning. It is enough. The hand that was halfway through the window to steal the mobile phone is hastily withdrawn and the two accomplices make off.

A few yards on we report the incident to a group of immaculately clad, on-duty unisex police. But the afternoon is warm, the news is inconvenient, and we are received with the empty face of official indifference.

On our arrival at Plaza de Acho the anti-bullfighting protest at the entrance is muted and good-natured. Everyone has played before, it's like an Old Boys' reunion.

'*¡Olé! ¡Olé!*' chant back *los aficionados* in rhythm with the protesters.

Nobody gets upset. We hand in our tickets and admire the old colonial structure, including El Mirador de Ingunza, a baroque folly built overlooking the bullring when supposedly the Viceroy, *El Virrey*, banned Señor De Ingunza and his (presumably) voluptuous mistress from entry to the Plaza for some alleged or actual misdemeanour. That way the loving couple could still enjoy the proceedings from their vantage point. Now the tower is in need of restoration before it collapses and steals away the evidence of this whimsical legend.

Less likely to collapse is *El cerro de San Cristobal*, the hill to the north-east of the Plaza, covered with matchbox dwellings in pastel greens, yellows, blues and pinks surmounted by a large cross and a billowing Peruvian flag.

The Doctor maintains an informative running commentary throughout the opening parade of *los toreros*, the bullfighting cast, with everyone resplendent in *nuevos trajes de luces*, shining new 'suits of lights'. *Los alguaciles*, the two sheriffs, lead the procession and the *matadores* themselves are of course well to the fore. Amongst the supporting roles, *los subalternos*, come *los picadores* mounted on their well-protected horses.

'Their job,' I am reminded, 'is to provoke the bull so that everyone can see just how furious he can be.'

No one is going to spoil a nice sunny afternoon by saying anything more on the subject of picadors, a necessary part of the ritual but there under sufferance. Like football referees, a hard-working, nicely presented, earnest body of men. But unloved, and nobody speaks to them at tea at the end of the afternoon. Picadors: one of life's little sadnesses. Even on those rare occasions when horse and rider get spectacularly overturned by a particularly ferocious bull, sympathy is not forthcoming from the crowd; the plaudits invariably go to *el toro*.

Next come *los monosabios*, the inexplicably named wise monkeys, an altogether different band of stalwarts, asking for nothing, expecting nothing and possibly even hearing nothing, dressed in red, white and black outfits. Their task is to remove successive dead bulls from sight, which they do more or less efficiently with the aid of three more or less obedient mules. Indeed, once the luckless bull has been harnessed and gathers speed across the arena, the *monosabios*, the mules and their cargo, disappearing from sight, resemble an escorted sand plough on carnival day.

The final unsung hero of the hour is *el arenaro*, the sandman and his wheelbarrow, befittingly bringing up the rear of the procession.

Today all three matadors come from Spain. The bulls also come from Spain: Dueno, Ratito, Adobado, Bapuleado, Novedoso and Famoso. As the Doctor explains, 'They put the name of the mother to the bull and then they are killed one by one according to age.'

And then the *monosabios* do the necessary.

*

73

The programme progresses. Dueno is despatched and in comes Ratito, closely followed by the first real surprise of the afternoon. Just once in a while the crowd likes to demonstrate its sense of fair play, and with no forewarning but with one accord, suddenly gives the picador a clap for deft work. He is naturally taken aback, but manages to maintain his phlegmatic composure. The matador is even more astounded when, living dangerously, he is subjected to two enormously high tosses from Ratito, happily without damage. Just a little dust on the new suit. But enough is enough. Curtains for the rash Ratito. A trophy of one ear, *una oreja*, is awarded by the judges to the *torero valiente*, brave and bruised. One of the sheriffs is pleased to make the presentation and the matador is showered with carnations, applause, sombreros, *botas de vino*, those leather wine carriers.

There are more surprises in store. The next bull, Adobado, is overcome with stage fright and has to be returned to the corral on the grounds of 'lack of force'. But now the offender is seized with a sudden burst of indignation and is reluctant to leave, least of all to go back up the tunnel.

Ready for just such an eventuality, a herd of six more bulls is introduced into the ring. Unfortunately, and in spite of the stern ministrations of a herdsman with a king-size cracking rawhide whip, they all mill around aimlessly, whilst the renegade bull sulks and petulantly throws his not inconsiderable weight of some 500 kilograms against anything and everything and refuses to associate with the new group. The reason for this quickly becomes apparent as, to make matters worse, the unruly newcomers choose to reveal strong hormonal desires and set about engaging in a little casual afternoon buggery, the worst of the gang blatantly rampant.

Los conocedores are spellbound and silent. Even the Doctor. The situation is fast getting out of hand. A second whipper-in appears, an *arriero* with a big *chicote*, to no avail. The gay group take a break from their activities and charge, sending all and sundry scuttling for cover. Fortuitously, this is the signal for the original troublemaker to trot calmly up the tunnel and the heavy wooden gate is banged triumphantly shut. Rather over-looking the fact that the gay group are still in the ring.

The crowd appreciates the diversion, but eventually it comes to an end. For a fleeting sacrilegious moment it appears that perhaps bullfighting, like motor racing, is one of those so-called sports that are only really interesting when things go wrong. No doubt such contaminated thinking is born of ignorance.

The imported tradition of bullfighting is historically part of the Peruvian tapestry; for the visitor the bullfight experience is a necessary one. The Doctor sums things up.

'In life,' he explains, 'you need to learn that everything that comes, it goes.' He pauses to gather his thoughts before con-tinuing. 'And everything that goes, comes first.'

The band plays on confidently and as a customary prelude to the sixth and final *corrida* the graceful *Marinera*, the dance of northern Peru, is presented in each entrance to the packed stands, adding yet more colour and activity to the busy scene.

'There are many variations,' the Doctor explains. 'The *Tondero* is more rapid; the version with no shoes owes more to the fields and less to the salons.'

'They are the laziest band in the southern hemisphere,' my neighbour declares with authority.

I have no way of knowing, but it seems possible.

'This music doesn't sound too well,' comments La Señora disapprovingly.

But as the Doctor has already reminded us, what comes, goes. A cool breeze fills the Plaza and dusk falls.

The following Sunday we do it all over again. The good lunch, this time at Casa Juan, *restaurante español*, preceded by that indispensable Peruvian aperitif, pisco sour.

'Here in Lima you make the appetite in the streets, then you eat in the house,' La Señora informs us enigmatically. But we are all agreed.

'It was a beautiful lunch.'

'*Sí*, very beautiful.'

We take our seats in the uppermost tier of the Plaza in time for the procession.

'Is La Señora coming?' ask our neighbours.

'Yes, she is coming very fast.' And indeed she appears, carrying a bottle of sherry, packed in a bag of CDs for some obscure reason.

'Has she a player?' ask the neighbours. 'No? Maybe it is a musical bottle.'

Maybe she has invented a new cooling device using deep-frozen CDs. The Doctor has his large cigar and is beaming, but is strangely quiet.

'La Señora has done a very good job quietening him,' I am informed in a whisper.

In fact, she has told him quite severely that he is 'like a merchandise person selling potatoes on the corner'. He is mutely obedient but undeterred and is still armed with a piercing whistle, a gift from heaven secretly envied by us all. This he deploys at unexpected moments, outwitting La Señora with a hint of ventriloquy, gazing steadfastly into the centre of the Plaza the whilst. But the beam is just a little bit broader.

And so the events of the afternoon unfold. The lumbering bulls and the agile matadors come and go, and with an increasingly experienced eye I believe that amongst the bewildering sequences of moves I detect possibly *una larga cambiado* followed by *una larga afarolada de rodillas*, a *derechazo de rodillas*, a *natural* and a *volapie*. But I couldn't swear to it. Anyway, it all merits much applause, acknowledged by the *torero*.

'Now he gives the bull time to breathe,' explains my adviser, in case I might be thinking of things the other way round.

In due course, with the sun low in the early evening sky, the programme is all but complete and all is well with the world. Except for our friend the picador. Until now he has enjoyed an uneventful day, suffering a minimum of abuse. He discharges his business with the final bull without provoking the crowd and heads thankfully for the exit, homeward bound. Presumably even picadors have a wife and family waiting for them after work. Then suddenly the bull makes a vengeful attack on unsuspecting horse and rider, completely justified but contrary to all the rules and norms of conduct. The picador is forced against his will to jab away with *la puya* in self defence, much to the vociferous indignation of the spectators. He retreats from view up the tunnel, a broken man. Bad luck really.

And there it is. All over for another week.

On arrival at Plaza de Acho you can buy a foam cushion to assist your greater comfort and enjoyment during the afternoon's entertainment. They cost one nuevo sol, or possibly two (or more) for gullible foreigners. It is best to buy an extra cushion for La Señora, who claims not to need one ('She has many cushions,' advises an anonymous voice from the back of the group), although once into the bullring it is a different story. Not only are the cushions a good investment but you get the simple pleasure of spinning them into the Plaza at the end of the day. Everybody does it, but I am humbled to receive a caution, like a yellow card, from La Señora.

'I never saw a Britishman do such a thing,' she says frowningly.

It is enough. I won't do it again.

Today we did not bring the car, the traffic is too tedious even with Rafael at the wheel ('I went to a British school, God save the King!'). La Señora takes charge of our group and leads the way to a waiting coach.

'Leave it to the Queen to ring the bells,' she tells us.

77

She is an expert sampler of street stalls, so we pause to buy *picarones* (fresh cooked fritters in syrup) and *anticuchos* (kebabs made from 'the heart of the beef from that very afternoon').

One of the curiosities of *las corridas* is the perceived necessity for the matadors to give a formal interview after the event for the benefit of *los aficionados*. It happens, so we go. The drive takes us through the Rimac area, run-down, unwashed, dusty and dangerous, just a few scant rungs superior to shanty town. As ever, La Señora and the Doctor are assiduous guides.

'Here they change the down part of your shoe for just five soles,' La Señora tells me.

I think about the unfortunate pile of pieces that were my favourite desert boots. At one pound it would have been a bargain.

'We just passed the prison,' says the Doctor. 'Now it is the police station. So you see how things are. Not much change. And this here is the live chickens' market.'

The coach arrives at the Country Club. Five stars, maybe six.

'Now in the hotel they are receiving us with hungry eyes,' observes La Señora shrewdly.

We join the press briefing. The main room is crowded, the bull-groupies to the fore, so we sit outside.

'Here is more fresh,' La Señora says with satisfaction.

Robbed of the glamour of their elaborate costumes, *los matadores* appear almost as ordinary mortals, but the audience reverently hangs on every word as they tell us how it was for them. No one asks how it was for the bulls.

Castellano is a language of many words, many nuances, conducive to flatulence. After an hour or two we feel the need to go home. But La Señora is right.

'It is bad education to leave in this moment,' she reminds us. 'It is not possible to go at this time of the hour.'

So we wait to the end and promise all our friends that we

will see them next week. Even if only to reflect on the similarities between bullfighting and endeavouring to succeed with a new maternity clinic.

'It is a complex dialogue between life and death,' explains the Doctor.

Exactly.

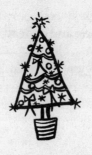

9

La Señora Peruana y Navidad

Christmas comes early to Lima. As it does to most of Peru, where to a greater or lesser extent Catholicism has joined uncritical hands with more ancient rituals, particularly high in the Andes and in the depths of the forests. For a full six weeks and more we are in the inescapable smothering grip of Navidad, that cheerfully permissive blend of Christianity and pagan festivals. However, it is a joyful time, as well it should be.

'This Clinic is a happy place,' declares La Señora, countenancing no possibility of contradiction. 'Here you see happiness in every corner.'

You do. All year round the routine is happily unchanging. Diminutive Nurse Dulce daily records the appointments, painstakingly marking the big diary with that slow, round hand of hers. In turn, the Doctor ministers to the varying needs of the visiting ladies, real, imagined, and unexpected, with the receptive inscrutability of long experience and with kind and understanding ear, while down below on the ground floor offhand Ernestina reluctantly dons her heavy horn spectacles in the office-under-the-stairs and takes the fees in the event that they are offered or makes a note on the lengthening list when they are not. Strapping Señorita Hilda strides sternly to and fro with her sheaves of important documents and behind the scenes on the fourth floor the imported adviser grapples with the sombre figures and forecasts that prognosticate certain doom, and head in hands looks enviously out across the gardens to the happy doves cavorting in the dead tree. Then he makes a mental note to ask La Señora yet again to curtail the shopping trips that daily fill the Clinic with those glorious but unnecessary bouquets of fresh flowers from Huaraz and Ecuador and that fleetingly line the shelves of our *cafetería* with an irresistible display of cherry-topped cream horns, walnut whirls and tempting truffles from the nearby *pastelería* which unaccountably vanish without trace long before the day is out.

We are indeed 'a home from home for the ladies'. Especially at Christmas time, when the decorations are up with November scarcely into its stride. (La Señora finds an excuse to decorate the Clinic in most seasons. Soon we will need a separate store for Halloween items, for giant Easter eggs and yellow chickens, Mothers' Day, Disney World, as well as all the trappings of Christmas.) There is a shop in Lima dedicated solely to Navidad, year round. Unfortunately, it is close to the Clinic and for La Señora it is another home from home.

'They make so much money selling happiness,' she tells us. True. Quite a lot of it was hers. The money, that is.

Somewhat surprisingly, we limit ourselves to three Christmas trees. Two in the Clinic, one in Casa Bonomini. All are works of art, the huge one in Casa Bonomini especially so. Ribbons and bows, golden heralds and silver cherubs adorn every cornice, every possible architectural protuberance throughout the Clinic. Our alpine cuckoo clock, a gift to the Doctor from a grateful patient and now mounted in Reception, can hardly function for the weight of decorative baubles, the labouring bird scarcely able to emerge to pronounce each passing hour, so that Nurse Dulce has to climb on a chair periodically to resuscitate the mechanism. In one of the downstairs bow windows we have a seated Father Christmas nodding and reading by the flickering fireside; in the other curved window we have waving teddy bears singing carols under lamplights.

The maze of wiring in support of all these illuminations is akin to the proverbial epileptic snakes' honeymoon and at this time of year the Doctor is traditionally diverted from his normal prenatal preoccupations to set everything in order rather than setting everything truly alight, but it is not his strongest suit.

'In this business of being the Christmas electrician, I am not so good,' he admits, shaking his head sadly and surveying the serpentine tangle before him. Notwithstanding, in the gloom of the misty evenings children come with their neatly starched nannies to gaze in at our windows, like a scene from Dickens, but without the snow. If they are lucky, and many are, then La Señora, Lady Bountiful personified, appears as if by magic and gives each child a colourfully wrapped present, even though there is at times some uncertainty as to the precise contents. Hopefully a cuddly toy but possibly a slightly inappropriate cookery book or a bottle of even more inappropriate Chanel Number 5 or something considerably stronger. Good for children to learn early on that life is a lottery, even at Christmas time.

La Señora returns from one of her frequent forays to the Christmas shop carrying a large box of reindeer antlers. Unfortunately there are enough for everyone, one set of antlers each.

'Do you have the character to wear these?' she demands to know.

'Yes of course,' we insist rashly.

Answer in haste, repent at leisure. No sooner are we all bedecked in the horns, than she has a further brainwave.

'In this moment, God bright me!'

More tinsel. For the antlers. We refrain from admiring the blushing red seasonal Ho! Ho! Ho! socks that La Señora is wearing. None of us has the character to wear antlers and tinsel and Ho! Ho! Ho! socks. She also has some Jingle Bells socks but we try not to think about them. Christmas can be a stressful time. Indeed, La Señora develops a new allergy.

'I am allergic to my office,' she declares, with absolute finality.

Season of goodwill and we are the target of an attempted robbery. It is not the first. Three well-dressed ladies arrive. Their mother (or was it their grandmother?) has an appointment with the Doctor, she will arrive in a moment, her name is in the book. We always offer new patients a tour of the Clinic. Perhaps later, they reply. They ask Nurse Dulce where the cashier is situated. Ernestina is under the stairs, she explains, ever helpful. We are delighted if patients pay in advance. Suddenly, and in the nick of time, the penny drops. For us, that is. Obvious really, with 20–20 hindsight. The well-dressed birds take fright and fly empty-handed, into a waiting car. Granny's name is false; we have the car details. Everything is passed to the police. We never hear another thing. Peace on earth.

The world undergoes its annual December transformation. In the local gymnasium, my refuge from the Clinic, personal trainers I have never met before are suddenly anxious and concerned for the amount of weight on my barbell and it is obvious that, given half a chance and without a second bidding, they would complete all my exercises by proxy. I am prompted to wonder if La Señora might be persuaded to harness some of this surplus energy for use in the Clinic gymnasium. Our *cartero*, postman and *portador de nuestra correspondencia*, emerges from anonymity by way of a colourful Christmas card, brimming with Faith and Hope and Prosperity. Especially the last.

The Clinic itself is alive with music and movement, carols and conversation. Happy families. An appointment with the Doctor is first and foremost a social event and, on those rare occasions when it is necessary, La Señora introduces patients to one another and proudly conducts tours of the Clinic. Ensconced in my office, I am aware of each group's arrival at the fourth floor. 'And this is where he sleeps,' explains La Señora, indicating my room at the end of the passage. There follows a respectful hush.

Normally in Peru conversations never end. Sometimes a gathering may shake hands, kiss emotionally and start to take their leave. But nobody really means it, nobody believes in the finality of the moment. Someone will make a remark or throw in a new topic and the situation is saved. Everyone settles down again, relieved and contented, talking simultaneously as before, nobody listening. Should anyone so forget themselves as to importunately exclaim 'oh-is-that-the-time-I-really-must-be-going' or any similarly intrusive sentiment such as expressing agreement with the speaker, thereby hazarding the prospect of eternal discussion, then they are studiously ignored until they return to their rightful senses and recover their composure.

Maybe these Peruvians are just practising their Castellano, everybody says you need to do that. Yes, that must be it. Even if you have the French and the Latin it needs daily practice. La Señora has fashioned her whimsical Victorian tea-room with the abundance of chocolate cakes and pastries to assist that very process of animation. If she didn't have such long and entwining Swedish roots she would have created an even more extensive English heritage. In solid oak. Either way, a visit to the Clinic is an event to be savoured, an occasion for chatting, for lingering. Especially at Christmas time.

*

84

In acknowledgement of the impending Millennium, and with a keen eye for marketing, La Señora is moved to institute the instant tradition of an annual photograph of our distinguished Doctor sitting amidst all his mums, new-borns and reluctant fathers. Generously there is even a chair for me, although my credentials are tangential rather than direct. The Doctor facetiously suggests that I might fill the post of Pregnancy Co-ordinator but La Señora, busy orchestrating the event and in no mood for levity, suggests otherwise.

For the Photograph of the Century, all the Doctor's eligible families from the past thirty or so years are invited to participate. The garden is crammed with people; there is hardly room for the plants. Dr Hermogenes wears his best tie for the portrait and a bemused expression. 'How did this happen?' he is asking himself as he surveys the multitude. 'Is this all my doing?' In due course La Señora peruses the freshly printed results of the assembly with satisfaction.

'In this picture,' she muses, 'the Doctor is more nearly handsome.'

A giant framed enlargement is ordered to decorate the entrance hall.

The photograph is a festive occasion. We are in our antlers and tinsel, except for La Señora, who, for reasons known only to her regal self, has opted for her Minnie Mouse ears. Predictably unpredictable at all times ('The inexpectable is more interesting, don't you think?').

Amidst the throng, shady Hortencio and dubious Portencio appear, also unexpectedly. Yes, of course we remember them, the shifty building *Obermeisters*, now decked in their Sunday best, dusty overalls discarded. Greetings are exchanged, the universal catechism of the courtesies runs its course.

'You owe us three thousand dollars,' pronounce Portencio and Hortencio in unison.

'¿*Qué?*' says Minnie Mouse, solo, upset.

I take off my antlers and tinsel. I need a clear head.

'Leave this to me,' I hear myself say. Whoosh! Minnie Mouse has gone. Why did I have to say that?

Of course we must pay all outstanding amounts, I assure the builders. From scrutiny of our records (what records?), I tell them, I had concluded that the account had been settled in full. But of course, I will re-check. If we are in error, obviously we must pay the arrears. Perhaps, I ask politely, they would be kind enough to do the same. Check their records, I mean. Let us meet again at eight o'clock in the morning on New Year's Day and see how we stand, so to speak, bringing our documentation to the table. Hortencio and Portencio nod, uncertainly. Oh yes, I go on, while you are here, would you be kind enough to come and see one or two points of detail that require your attention? This roof, for example . . .

We never see Hortencio and Portencio again. There must have been an oversight in their documentation. Peace on earth. Perhaps, after over half a century, I am beginning to learn one or two of the lessons of life. I put my antlers back on, and the tinsel. Now, where has Minnie Mouse gone?

Christmas Eve and we prepare red-ribboned hampers for the staff. Fruit, chocolates, Italian *panetone*, Spanish *biscocho*, sweet bread and currants. And a 6kg turkey apiece. Everybody is pleased, especially white-haired ancient Manolo, our new security guard. In all his many years of previous service he has never before had a hamper, so he is prompted to make an involuntary but moving expression of appreciation and then overflows with the unendurable emotion of the occasion. We avert our eyes as his wrinkled little face contorts to control the huge tears that splash wetly on to the exquisite white timbers of the auditorium floor with every shuddering sob and I wonder if I am alone in being concerned lest the deluge might cause those fine floorboards, imported at such expense from distant parts, to warp beyond repair, causing in turn yet more distortion to our stress-filled finances. But, as always, La Señora is equal to the occasion. 'Don't cry,' she exclaims, 'here, eat something!'

And Manolo disappears from sight, enveloped in the warmest of Yuletide hugs.

As *vigilantes* go, Manolo is not really a big man. In fact, he is about four foot six. When he was younger he may have been taller, perhaps four foot seven, but now that he is three score years and ten and a little bit more, he is a little bit less, in a manner of speaking. Manolo has an imposing shiny-peaked cap and an equally shiny uniform for his doorstep duties and is a favourite with our clientele. Like something out of a Christmas cracker. He has the rare ability to sleep standing up, unsupported, heron-like. Wily fox that he is, his cap is three sizes too large so that his eyes are well covered. When Manolo is sleeping he sways gently from side to side; fortunately the wind never blows too strongly in Lima. Maybe he too went to medical school in his youth, although it seems unlikely. From dusk to dawn he has a little sentry box on wheels, ordained and arranged by La Señora, and at the setting of the sun he takes his place therein and sleeps soundly through the night in direct contravention of his orders. Not for him 'the watchman's steady tread in the silent dark'. One of these long nights the pixie box will surely roll away down the slope, taking Manolo with it, never to be seen again, back to toytown whence he came.

But just at this moment he can hardly manage to carry his struggling Christmas hamper. 'Next year,' Señorita Hilda tells him sternly, 'we will have to give you a lighter turkey.' At this he looks anxious and redoubles his efforts. He is a determined man and eventually he totters off triumphantly down the road from the Clinic, encouraged and supported by Nurse Dulce and goaded by giggling Ernestina. Thus it is that we go our separate ways for the festivities, everyone fondly exchanging the Season's Greetings yet again.

In Casa Bonomini La Señora arranges an extravaganza for the Eve of Christmas. This is the signal for the maid to leave. She just goes, no words, no farewell. Like a sunset without a sunrise. Gone for ever. It is the way.

'Because of this maid, my liver grows,' complains the mistress of the household.

'Oh, you lost your maid!' cry La Señora's sympathetic friends, secretly enjoying less charitable thoughts. 'Worse than losing a husband!'

Definitely, but never mind, we have others. Maids, that is. It's a mere hiccup and La Señora's party juggernaut is shock-proof and armour-plated.

'I used to have a second maid,' she tells us, 'but she was too friendly with the *chofer* and when she became pregnant I decided the family was growing too large. Now I am happy in my house alone with my turkey.' We nod understandingly. 'Sometimes I am an executive person, sometimes I can be an *ama de casa*, a housewife. I like to do the breads for Christmas myself and for my house to smell of baking. My other old maid Robbery Rosario will return to help me. If she wants to rob everything she will do. We were missing a little bit of her touch. She steals a lot but she cooks deliciously.' This last comes as an afterthought as though it is Robbery Rosario herself who is going into the oven and not the turkey.

In reality the extravaganza is something of a Yuletide waifs and strays party. Extended family, of course. *Noblesse oblige*. All the distant relatives catch up on the news. The juicy snippets are tossed busily to and fro, and fragments flutter in the night air like hovering moths. 'He is warming the tea pot and watering the broccoli,' a voice explains. Eyes open wide and knowing looks are exchanged. 'She is a very conflicted person, it seems that she is not too well recognized by the rest of the group,' comes another snippet, and mysteriously, 'There was an awful row in that, bim-bam-bum, it was a bad image to society.' Or less mysteriously, 'He had nine children and three more outside the house.' And 'Is she married?' answered by 'No, she just had some children by some men here and there.'

Will the night be long enough to cover all the activities of these busy brethren, we ask ourselves? Possibly not, the exchange of information is in full flow now. 'She is younger in body than his other wife, of course. But when I saw them, he was walking behind, wallet ready in the pocket, not with a happy face. Of course, she is just the most recent wife of this man.' It seems the agenda is very full this year. 'He put his feet out of the pot, he looked for other butterflies and he was kicked off, then he cried *cocodrilo* tears. Ha! He thought he was the top of the cake.' It is without end. Gossip: truly one of the most powerful forces in the universe.

Then there is the legacy of the Russians. A few years ago La Señora the artist found fame, if not fortune, when she was invited to display her alluring canvases in Moscow. The invitation was founded on the professional merits of her assorted contorted naked nymphs, of course, but there may have been undertones, or overtones. Possibly. Probably. Hence the Russian legacy at the Yuletide party. People with obvious cover names, such as Boris, Alexi, Dmitri and Igor, and silent wives with watchful eyes, startlingly blond, impenetrably coiffured. Like Prancer and Dancer and the rest of the crew, they are never seen from one end of the year to the other, only on Christmas Eve. Strange that I should come all the way to Peru to spend La Nochebuena with Russians. But as one does with

Russians, we chat about the usual topics, James Bond and John Le Carré, Inov the Red the Siberian snooker ace, general Bolshoi and so forth. Lots of nudging and winking and everyone remembers to laugh. Loud and long. Ah, we sigh, catching our breath, if only it wasn't for that revolution. How fine things could have been.

On this occasion the Russians have reinforcements to hand; conveniently a trade delegation is in town. They join the party and we circle the newcomers with menacing hospitality in our Father Christmas hats with the moose ears. The guests eye us warily, scanning unsuccessfully for the microphones and hidden cameras. To add piquancy to the occasion La Señora is using her Mata Hari-style cigarette holder, whilst the Doctor, courteous as ever and obviously not wishing to be outdone, helpfully introduces me as 'our contact with MI6'. The effect is electric: eyes pop, jaws drop.

'He has a black joke style,' says La Señora, by way of clarification, casually flicking ash on to the carpet.

'*¿Más champaña, caballeros?* More champagne, gentlemen?' enquires the Doctor smoothly, popping another cork and emptying another bottle. He blows a nonchalant wish into the magnum, as is the custom, and seals it with his hand. I guess that he is dreaming of horses again. Or great big bulls.

'Be careful with your drinks please,' cautions La Señora, casting a firm glance in the Doctor's vicinity and then swivelling unexpectedly like a circling condor to catch me in her sights. 'After drinks you become changed persons.'

'My tongue shall be as a silver bell from heaven,' promises the Doctor, living dangerously. Someone starts to snigger, but the condor swiftly puts a stop to that.

As the reassuring champagne is poured I take advantage of the diversion and yawn widely to capture a quick panoramic snap of the guests with the camera implanted in my wisdom tooth, upper right (occlusal filling). Nice shot, I tell myself, HQ should be pleased. Sometimes after a good dinner the lens can get a bit smudged with gravy or even obscured by a slice of carrot or a lettuce leaf, and the message from Moscow ends up with an unexpected chicken or garlic flavour, but I sense that this time there were no such technical hitches. Perhaps a little heavy on the turkey and *panetone* sponge cake in the foreground but still good. As a decoy I pass my Box Brownie to Uncle Anastacio visiting from Florida and he does the necessary. The Russians are edgy so smilingly I put them at their ease.

'One copy for London, one for Moscow.'

Everyone relaxes. Fair's fair. The older Russian in the well-cut suit that has to have been made in the west, even Savile Row, speaks Spanish. The younger Russian in the white shirt and no suit speaks French. The middle-aged Russian in the double-breasted people's shiny sack suit laughs charmingly but says nothing.

'What second language does your charming friend speak?' I ask the Savile Row Russian.

'English. He speaks English. But it is not so active.'

'Ah.' All suits are equal but some suits are more equal than others.

Not forgotten are that small and exclusive band of supporting medical practitioners who have with astute hopefulness connected themselves to the Clinic. They are dutifully invited to the party, plus any handy spouses in the hope of brightening and further enlivening the evening. For La Señora, doctors are a necessary and lovable breed of many talents, none greater than their potential, both individually and collectively, to be a major disorganization. Perhaps on account of those long years of arduous study. Perhaps the human brain has a finite capacity, like a computer. Put too much in and something falls out.

Take Dr Desastre. As with the itinerant mender of pots and pans, *el jilguero* of Miraflores, he is an inexplicable favourite with La Señora, unfathomable as always.

'We have a wonderful young nutritionist who specializes in putting people in and out,' she informs the world at large and anyone else who happens to be passing, as is her wont.

Be that as it may, in the autumn the miraculous young nutritionist, he of the eat-as-much-as-you-like regimes of popular acclaim, was visited by his brother from afar, so a Casa Bonomini banquet was prepared and consumed in their honour. The dinner went well, but without Dr D. and his visiting brother. They arrived some three hours later, slightly flustered. That at least was to their credit. The table was heavy with fine wines and brandy, but to punish them it was insisted they try the nutritional virtues of non-alcoholic Chicha Morada, '*la bebida de los Incas*', made from purple maize and excellent for the brain. Until the hint of a tremble in Dr D.'s lower lip dictated that the sentence should be hastily remitted to avoid an embarrassing scene and the offenders were poured something with fewer vitamins but greater fortification. Crisis averted, we settled happily to a second feast.

However, that was not the end of it. When Dr Desastre was going on vacation, a *fiesta de despedida* was convened at Casa Bonomini. But Dr D. never made it to his farewell party, not at all. He must have been busy with the last-minute packing.

For the evening Yuletide gathering of waifs and strays he gives things an original twist. He comes for lunch. Incredible. Not just early, not just late, not just not at all. He comes for lunch: the wrong meal, half a day in advance. Freshly pressed shirt, freshly trimmed tonsure. Touching really. Probably fresh aftershave as well, but I refrain from checking. La Señora and Dr Hermogenes are the epitome of Peruvian hospitality. There, in a trice, is the waiting place at the table, no hint of surprise, not an indication given, not a word is said. Dr Desastre talks unconcernedly as he watches with satisfaction the preparations for his repast. Assuredly he will never learn that life is for listening.

The other doctors, with their more or less enlivening wives, assemble correctly for the party later in the day. Dr Cleeber is punctual to the minute, mingling thoughtfully, appraising the cosmetic possibilities on offer and mentally sharpening his scalpel. The chuckling Chinaman, Dr Ching, deposits his sandwich box in the hall along with his coat, hopeful that at the end of the party there may be a good selection of chocolates and petits-fours remaining to scoop into the plastic specimen container but meantime determined to enjoy the occasion to the full. Thus he compensates for the more circumspect and introverted demeanour of menopausal Dr Vonday, who finds Christmas a difficult time. An even more difficult time than usual, that is. And what of Dr D., the balding fringe man and world-class diaryless disorganizer? Yes, he comes too; by chance this unmissable event is writ large in some corner of his unreliable memory. Maybe he was just hungry at lunchtime and happened to drop by.

The honour of being Papá Noel falls to the unsuspecting newcomer. Me. There is a shortage of volunteers and an absence of snow in Lima, nothing deep or crisp or even. It is uncomfortably hot in the beard and big boots. Part of the established performance involves climbing out of one of the bedroom windows on to the Casa Bonomini verandah roof, tossing presents to the younger members of the extended family, gathered excitedly and expectant on the lawn below. By mistake I nearly follow the presents off the roof down into the waiting crowd. Not so much because of the excellence of the champagne, you understand, but because my glasses steam up. But no one believes me and I may not get the invitation to perform again next year. No words are spoken, but I sense that my position is being considered. Thankfully. It will be a merciful release. Not only that, Margarita, the enormous first-cook of African ancestry, insists on sitting on Papá Noel's knee for endless photographs, prompting warmly tactile memories and recollections of the two sacks of fine rice from Chiclayo.

Photo opportunity over, it is off in the big, once-white truck with my youthful entourage to dispense candy and good cheer to the neighbourhood children, most of whom went or were sent to bed long before our tardy arrival. Fortunately I have had the foresight to carry with me my traditional trombone to catch their attention. ('Are you rehearsalling your trombone?' La Señora has been asking me for days in advance.) Traditional? Well, it is now. Even so, we are so late doing our festive rounds that in some streets we merely succeed in disturbing the homeless sleeping on the pavements of up-market Miraflores who find themselves rudely awakened by a deluge of hard-boiled sweets falling from the star-lit heavens.

Driver of the truck is Medical Student Two, which is something of a mistake. He delights in cornering so fiercely that in the back we slide squealing hither and thither from side to side like hyperactive go-go girls. Co-pilot is Medical Student One, doubling as Candyman in charge of the bags of sweets, and fortunately possessed of a good embouchure, so he helps out with clarion calls on the trombone. And like all celebrities I have my stunt man in attendance, cousin-by-appointment Galolo, to stand in for the difficult bits, although goodness knows where he was when I was on, and almost off, the roof. I suspect that he has jealous ambitions to get the lead role in this pantomime. All things come to him who waits. For once that may prove true. However, now he makes amends for his earlier absence and with the novel aid of a balloon, as used (he says) by many a ventriloquist, he does Papá Noel's complete script of 'Ho! Ho! Ho!'s with commendable vigour and resonance.

We return to the Yuletide party hot and hoarse to find that La Señora, breaking with custom, has a surprise present for Papá Noel.

'This is your quotation,' she says, making the presentation. 'There, now the surprise is done.'

Surprise indeed. What a nice quota, a handsome bicycle. So many bicycles in my life; there has to be a message. There and then Medical Student Two, national motorcross junior champion (almost), offers to show me how to do a wheelie. He hides his disappointment well when I am forced to inform him that wheelies are not on my list of immediate ambitions and that for the time being two wheels will suffice thank you.

What's this? Another present? It is the time of giving. Maybe it's a little pot of grease for my new bike?

'No,' explains La Señora. 'This special cream is for the turkey neck. It will put your skin in a moment of renewal and make you shrinkle free.'

Gobble, gobble, wobble, wobble, turkey neck? Oh well, at least the kind thought is seasonal. '*Muchísimas gracias, Señora*, very kind indeed.'

'Very kind indeed?' repeats La Señora. 'I know that expression. That is the English push to the side.'

After the excitement and non-excitement I am pleased to untie the pillow from under my red jacket and to remove my whiskers, waving the while to the barman. Hilmutt is his name and I get him to repeat it, just to be certain. Curiously, Hilmutt has only one ear, with the other side of his head like an empty house with the window boarded.

'Where it is,' says the Doctor, referring to the missing ear, 'nobody knows.'

But apart from a certain lack of visual symmetry, it seems to make little difference. That's as long as you remember to place your order on his right side. Order on the left, and you have a long and thirsty wait. Hilmutt is at ease with the situation.

'*Feliz Navidad*, Hilmutt Cup-Head!' say his friends.

'Same to you,' he replies politely, 'Happy Christmas!'

Some time in the small hours long after midnight the invited, astutely hopeful doctors in turn give fine speeches of appreciation for everything in general and for nothing in particular.

But it falls to German Dr Vonday, specialist in matters menopausal, to give the ultimate and finest speech of all. The lateness of the hour lends poetry and pathos to his pronouncements and predictions and we find ourselves moved profoundly by the eloquence of his words. 'I was born in dark December,' he reveals, as though to lend weight to his seasonal oratory. 'Winter's child.' He pauses. Somehow we already knew that he was winter's child. 'My mother called me Tannenbaum, her little Christmas Tree.' We gaze upon Dr Vonday with new eyes. Little Tannenbaum in his mother's arms. He is full of late night hope. Von day, von day . . . everything vill be fine. But ve vonder. In the still of the enchanted silence La Señora's toy electric train, loaded with chocolates, whirrs solemnly round and round through the silver and crystal on the dining-room table, the candles flicker in the night air and everybody cries. Vonderful. Happy Christmas! Happy Christmas, Tannenbaum!

Christmas Day brings a rude awakening. At first I think it is the turkey and *panetone* making a fighting comeback, but then I decide it is an earthquake. The fourth floor of the Clinic wobbles like a jelly in the hands of an inebriated butler and I hold on to both walls simultaneously as previously instructed but fortunately nothing falls, not even my framed photo (unsigned) of one-time Manchester City goalkeeper Bert Trautman on the bedside table. Just a few crooked pictures. I look down out of the window and there are my neighbours sitting round their swimming pools. More compliments of the season. Just a tremor, they assure me. Oh good, just a tremor. Like a spot of indigestion. Nothing that need interrupt our enjoyment of Aunt Hermenegilda's excellent lunch later in the day. Until I spot the Doctor beckoning to me through the branches of the Christmas tree. I draw closer, curious.

'The race is at 4.30,' he whispers, part hidden by a scarlet cracker and a silver bell. I nod, uncomprehendingly. 'A thousand metres, Shessira and Big Bertha.'

I nod again, now I've got it. We slip out from Aunt Hermenegilda's merry gathering like two schoolboys playing truant, dodging the ever-rotating antenna of La Señora's early-warning radar, slide into the once-white truck and speed off to the racecourse, El Hipódromo de Monterrico with its stately sabres, the national tree of Venezuela.

The Doctor spots our new trainer.

'This man there is the trainer. He has a trouty face.'

It is true. Very fishy. Adolfo, the tiny elastic jockey, leaps aboard Big Bertha. He is about the same size as Manolo, our fearsome *vigilante*, but about half a century younger.

'Nice flanks,' I remark, knowledgeably.

The Doctor looks at me, taken by surprise.

'Bertha,' I explain. 'Big arse.'

The spirit of Mickey Moto, the departed Chinaman now vanished mysteriously to Miami, hovers over the racetrack, particularly in the shape of his bizarre flaming diamond racing colours. We also spare a warm thought for Mrs Moto in her nice short skirts. And we look lingeringly and longingly at the winner's enclosure. Maybe Papá Noel will oblige where others have failed.

But it is not to be. Shessira puffs home a gallant fifth, bringing in a handful of nuevos soles to put towards the feed. But not for two months. The cheque is post-dated. That's the way they do things at cash-strapped El Hipódromo. Cash flow management, that's what it's called. Unheard of in some quarters. As for Big Bertha with the fat flanks mounted by Adolfo the dwarf? Last. Plumb, unashamedly, last. Maybe next time. Indeed, on Boxing Day our gallant filly Expectativa races in for an exciting third place. *Poco a poco*, little by little. But for today, well, we drive back to Aunt Hermenegilda's in silence and it takes a while for us to pick up again on the merriment of the occasion.

Thus the high fever of another Christmas comes and goes. Season of prolonged anticipation and hope. Sometimes unfulfilled. However early you put up the decorations, Christmas always manages to catch you unawares. Off guard. Like rushing into a dark tunnel and then emerging blinking into the sunlight when it's all over, being caught by surprise, overtaken by events. A magical time of mixed emotions. Happy-sad. Remembered happiness, new-found sadness. Christmas is like that. Bittersweet. A time of reckoning for the inescapable normally invisible stealthy emotional burdens of a lifetime. Now, the brightness of the tinsel is fading, the lights on the tree are dimming. Taking down and packing away the decorations: the melancholy part of the festivities. Another year of life has slipped away.

'Christmas is only a difficult time for those who want to make it difficult,' declares La Señora briskly in her no-nonsense voice. 'If you want it to be a time of suffering, then suffer. Except always I find I have no time to unsemble the Christmas tree.'

In fact it is time to salute the summer that has now arrived in Lima, time to move down the coast to the beach house to greet the brave New Year, the beckoning New Millennium. Not that it is in our minds to abandon the Clinic. We can't. It needs us. And our patients need us. Equally, we need them. The equation is simple. To balance the books we must augment the numbers, but practically every month new theories with varying degrees of unconvincing implausibility are propounded to excuse our inability to advance: prospective clients are enjoying themselves at the seaside; now they are paying the school fees; now their taxes are due; now they have gone abroad; now once again Christmas is coming or has just gone and soon it will be Easter, ad infinitum. Nevertheless, the insomnolent reality, like the oft-told small cloud advancing on the horizon, no bigger than a man's hand, is that the Bank is threatening implacably. The grey-faced financiers are greedily eyeing the juicy goose, even without the golden eggs. Undeterred, and as ever blithely confident that tomorrow's problems may be entrusted to the morrow, Dr Vonday and the faithful toiling trio are primed to hold the fort and off we go, southwards to seek the sun. The New Millennium will surely herald new fortunes.

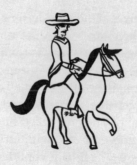

10

La Playa

So we say goodbye to our Christmas in Lima and the unfinished business of the Clinic, migrating southwards like swallows to the long golden beaches of Cañete with the long Pacific rollers and even longer days of golden sunshine. We endeavour to maintain our outward calm, but the New Year is upon us, heralded as in the entire globe with fireworks and dancing. For us it is the rhythms of the sustaining *salsa* and the mellifluous *merengue* from Cuba, Puerto Rico and Santo Domingo that see us into the early morning, that take us through the gates of the Third Millennium. With our 'hands on the future', we sing, we dance, we embrace. And, expectantly, we wait to be embraced by the twenty-first century.

To facilitate the transmogrification, La Señora follows custom, or superstition, eats twelve grapes for good fortune and then, wearing at least one garment in yellow, races breathlessly and theatrically round the beach house bearing a suitcase and a sprig of *ruda*, the good luck herb, to ensure that in the coming year she will travel safely, far and wide.

La Playa

The fireworks fade, the music dies. Only the most pedestrian of souls can be unmoved by the magic of the hour. Cautiously, exploringly, we wonder how we feel for this historic event, the advent of a new millennium. Something which has happened only once before since the birth of Christ.

'To this we will never return,' reflects La Señora. 'Forget the past, forget the future. Sense the present, know the hour, take the moment.'

We feel we should feel different but, a little disappointingly, we feel the same. *Así es la vida.* Thus is life. Our hearts are beating, it is enough. If the stroke of midnight had removed all the familiar landmarks, we would be lost, confused. Sufficient for the hour to sense the conflict of the old and the new.

'You can tell now that you lived a hundred years,' observes La Señora, somewhat surprisingly.

It is time to greet the New Millennium in wondering solitude, in silent contemplation, 'under the wide and starry sky'. That is the way for the blessed, the extrasensory, the telepathic to touch the fragility of the occasion. The Fourth Dimension. Permanent but transitory.

'I hope that life will give me a few more years,' says a familiar voice, softly, 'so that I may think on the future.'

We breathe deeply on the mystique of the Third Millennium. Under the Southern Cross and all those stars of the midnight sky that 'fill the mind with thoughts too big for words' we are joined by the symphonic tumble of those long Pacific rollers. Under the same wide sky, just a few hours earlier, kindred spirits thousands of miles away had shared a similar communion, but in the company of Ursa Major, the Plough and the Pole Star at Land's End, listening to the roar and crash of the wild Atlantic. Yes, this is the way to salute the New Millennium, in the open spaces of the planet, in the deserts, in the dark forests, in the majestic mountains, on the stretching shores of the vast oceans. In all the remote places of the globe. We thought to share the moment with Times Square, Trafalgar Square, Paris, Rio and all the other great cities of the world. But this is the way. In wondering quietness, in isolation, forgotten in a hidden corner of the universe. The caress of loneliness. The excitement of solitude. Yes, we hope that life will give us a few more years.

On New Year's Day we rise early, earlier than most, to breathe again the vibrance of the Third Millennium, to hear afresh the thundering symphony of the rolling waves. La Señora explains the evolution of the golden beach.

'The ocean frictions the stones and there you have the sand.'

The Doctor rolls his eyes in affirmation.

We are indeed in the minority; the vast majority are still sleeping their lives away. We share the dawn with the dishevelled leftovers from the excesses of the night before, subdued and straggling, homeward bound. One fiesta has yet to die. Tired laughter, the music of the night unequal to the light of day. Two youths fight, drunk or drugged, both or neither. Along the beach, in the intimate seclusion of the almost deserted expanse of sand, a bald fat man is kissing a woman, no longer young. He is interested, pressing. She stands, hands on hips as though she might be in a check-out queue at the supermarket, waiting for him to finish. 'Next customer please' reads the neatly printed sign on the conveyor belt. The brave new world of the Third Millennium. The gulf between reality and dreams; how it is and how we hope.

The summer sea is seducing us, in conflict with the call of the Clinic.

'I learnt from my Breetish,' declares La Señora, neatly putting the onus on me. 'At the weekends we are obligated to go to the beach.'

So we commute from Lima to Cañete, and back again, Cañete to Lima. South, north, south, north. South to the seaside, north to the city. Rarely do we escape from the Clinic on a Friday evening, and even then it is long after dark before we lock the doors and drive away to the sea; more usually we are forced to watch a hot and sunny Saturday fade into late afternoon before the intermittent stream of patients and other Clinic callers permit us to be on our impatient way. Sometimes we are tempted to delay our reluctant return to the city until Monday's uncertain dawn, then invariably agreeing in consequence that it would have been better to have returned on the Sunday night in preparation for the week ahead.

The Doctor's and La Señora's beach house is not the newest in Cañete; possibly it is the oldest and probably one of the smallest, certainly one of the noisiest and happiest. Everybody squeezes in and the only complaint comes from the plumbing.

'This is the room for our visitors,' is La Señora's greeting for all new arrivals, expected and unexpected alike. 'But first we have to pass the brush and sweep the dust.' Woe betide the guest who mistakenly leaves his bed during the night to answer the demands of nature. On return from the mission it is quite possible that the recently vacated haven will be in the possession of a foreign body. Hot-bunking happy families.

'Don't worry,' declares La Señora. 'If more people come, they can go in a hamcock.'

Oh yes, of course, a hamcock. Nobody ever knows how many people will arrive for the weekend. It all depends on who turns up.

'How many floors does your house have?' ask the neighbours, eyeing the bungalow curiously. 'We see so many people coming out.'

For three months we enjoy the non-culture of sun, sand and surf. Mainly serenaded by the sounds of music and laughter, less frequently we bask in the sound of silence so profound that a breakfast teaspoon in a breakfast teacup can be heard from a hundred metres.

Noisy or tranquil, a central figure in our beach existence is Abraham the butler, redeployed Clinic-cleaner and recycled *plaza* car-washer. Possessed of a voice like a rowing boat grounding on shingle, Abraham is an artillery veteran of the Peruvian armed forces. They trained him well. Day in, day out, he launches relentless assaults against dust and debris, real and imagined. The military in general do little, but what they do, they do early. Abraham certainly does things early, greeting the dawn with his gravel voice to ensure that everyone in the overfull beach house is conscious of just how promptly he is on parade, manning the front line whilst lesser mortals sleep, or try to. But atypically, he works late too. For Abraham the cleaning battle is unremitting, never ending. Truly a war without truces or prisoners. He wipes, washes, sweeps and shines from dawn to dusk, advancing at a steady steely-eyed pace, like the parson's vintage sit-up-and-beg one-speed bicycle proceeding through the village with the wicker basket in front. Unswerving, unnerving, the forces of cleanliness with godliness close at hand.

Once a month, with an artilleryman's precision, Abraham resigns. They say it is the Andean way.

'I refuse him,' states La Señora with matching precision. 'We need him.'

Abraham listens respectfully to the rejection of his request and carries on cleaning, no doubt making a mental note to try his luck again the following month. For he is made of stoical stuff and, like others, the driving force for his 'interior life' comes from his secret passion. His is not a life of quiet desperation. Abraham is from Ayacucho, key city in the Peruvian struggle for independence where 'on 9 December 1824 a mestizo force commanded by Marshal Sucre defeated the occupying army and effectively ended Spanish rule in Peru'. Ayacucho is also the heartland of *la danza de las Tijeras*, an energetic and traditional dance involving curious metal instruments with a resemblance to scissors. Abraham is a leading exponent of this colourful ritual of the Southern Andes that combines frog-swallowing with toad-tasting, cheek-piercing needles and cane spirit. As he brooms and brushes and clears for action, his inner being is surely dancing and jigging to the violin and the harp, secure in the care of the *wamani*, the spirit of the mountains.

Indeed, the summer beaches of Cañete are home to many passions. The canoeists who brave the surf to reach the off-shore islands to marvel at the dolphins, the seals, the penguins, the squadrons of pelicans and the flocks of smaller seabirds that sometimes pass, stretching from horizon to horizon. The volleyball players who endure the fierce glare of the midday sun to demonstrate that their sport is not a matter of life or death, but something beyond. The youthful surfers with their happy boards, immune to the chill of the Humboldt current, with or without El Niño and La Niña, who return home as the sun sets. They should be weary and waterlogged but instead they shake off the salt and the sand and prepare to dance the night away.

There are the sculptors in sand, sometimes erotic, sometimes not, who win generous prizes for their skills in competitions sponsored by our over-rich Bank. There are the eternal debaters of the beach, who ask for nothing more than an attentive audience, an unending stream of news and a fountain flowing with good gossip. There are the latter-day Incas, those worshippers of the Sun and Mother Earth, the inert and colourful confetti of the sands who seek only a cloudless sky. Whilst for those unequal to the challenge of the noontime heat, a few dozen nuevos soles buys the somnolent shade of a palm-thatched *sombrilla*, complete with the owner's name. 'Jhon Lemon' is what they write on my cool new sunshade, a memorial for years to come. Until wind and tide transform it into an epitaph.

On the water are the noisy jet skiers, an obese sport. Thankfully the drivers spend most of their day pushing and pulling their trailers through the sand, and then stand in busy huddles drinking beer from bottles, wearing goggles. It must be special, extra-fizzy beer. Also at the water's edge are the motionless surf gatherers, mystical beings with empty eyes poised silently at the ocean's end to hang the waves in their hands and catch the foam on their toes, in solitary communion with the great waters. They are distant figures on the shore, possessed of no one to oil their sunburnt shoulders: one of the great lonelinesses of life. That and having no one to catch the frisbee.

On the paved promenade are the zipping roller bladers, valiant gliders of the palm-fringed paving stones. Whilst in the air above the beaches the marketing men seize the day to hire light aircraft towing banners advertising grand stores such as Mr Wong's, with his soothing haemorrhoid cream and much more. D'Onofrio is up there too, tormenting us from every aspect, every angle, from land and air. Maybe soon the pilot will be blowing one of those *trompetas* as he passes. The indications are clear: preparations must be made to repel an amphibious invasion by the three-wheeled yellow peril as countless cold-boxes trundle relentlessly up the beaches, mating and multiplying as they come, *cornetitas* sounding 'Charge!' If that were not enough, even our bank manager invests in a banner. '*Feliz Ano Nuevo*' he says, as well he might, considering that we are paying the annual interest charges per anum. In his haste he has forgotten his *tilde*, the vital Castellano 'wiggle' in *Año*, but we forgive him, knowing that he means

Happy New Year even though he has vulgarly wished us something quite fundamentally different.

Then there is the secret society of 18-speed mountain bikers. They have a hidden code to ensure they all wear the same colour jerseys on any given day, and arrange their laundry accordingly. Nobody knows how they know. Perhaps it is a broken twig on the path, a sign with the left thumb when they drink their *luisa* herb Inca Cola and Cola Inglesa, a pull on the ear, even a snapped zinnia in the second flowerbed on the right. Nobody knows, the code is changed daily, the laundry unerringly arranged.

The secret society of mountain bikers has a special whistle to summon its members in the morning. 'Pee whee pee!' they call to each other, 'pee whee pee!' 'Come-a-long, come-a-long!' Then they move to a minor key to thwart frivolous and confusing impostors, such as the mischievous Doctor. 'Pee pee whee whee!' they whistle. 'Hurry up with your breakfast!'

'Pee whee pee,' answers the Doctor, dodging into the creamy pendulous depths of an adjacent Angel's Trumpet tree, grinning like a gleeful peewit.

Our next-door neighbour, Biker Rafo, is always late with his breakfast. The other bikers congregate outside his house, and ours, impatient, eager to be off. Cough, cough, cough they go, come along Rafo! Finally the door of the house opens slowly and reluctant Rafo's dutiful wife, freshly warm from the conjugal bed, wheels out his sleepy bicycle and then wheels out her tardy husband. And off go the mountain bikers, whirring through life like partridges with eighteen complicated gears, heads down, bottoms up. The local *campesinos*, the country folk, watch with wide-eyed curiosity.

'What are they doing?' the residents ask each other wonderingly.

'They like to be tired,' comes the explanation.

'Oh . . . *Sí*.'

The bikers have special shoes, special paradoxical gloves without fingers and special go-faster banana shorts. With the help of this wondrous technology they can levitate into the surrounding hills to inaccessible vantage points, to be met (to their infinite surprise) by the ubiquitous yellow-coated D'Onofrio man wearing flip-flop slaps, with his own irritating whistle and no special gloves, baggy second-hand Florida shorts and his one-speed yellow ice box on wheels, full of refreshing ice cream.

The elegant riders of *los caballos de paso peruanos*, the evocative Peruvian pacing horses, the very epitome of culture-casted Peru, also journey into the hills behind the beaches of Cañete, sombreros tilted against the sun, ponchos flowing. Yes, surely the very essence of Peru, *los embajadores silenciosos* as they call them, the graceful pacing horses, the silent ambassadors, are descendants of the Andalucian and Berber mounts that accompanied the first conquistadors to South America in the sixteenth century. With their genetically inherited trotting style they move their feet in pairs on the same side, one two, three four, instead of 'diagonally', one four, three two, like other horses. That's if you observe sufficiently attentively with a quick enough eye. No one is likely to contradict but it makes the difference between a stable platform for the rider and one that bounces and rolls. Ideal for novices. And a picture of unrivalled equine beauty, the lyrical inspiration of poets, musicians and artists alike.

Twice I am invited to ride *un caballo de paso*. Once at sunrise to journey into the mountains overlooking the distant white surf-fringed sands of *la costa*, beyond the reach of the secret society of 18-speed bikers and the whistling yellow D'Onofrio irritant in his regular slaps and baggy shorts. And once at dusk, after a bull-branding barbecue on one farm, when we ride through the eucalyptus trees to a neighbouring hacienda for further refreshment. Wearing my hand-stitched blue shirt with the inadvertent short sleeves, tailor-made for barbecues. *Los caballos de paso peruanos*: those balletic Peruvian steeds, internationally coveted.

The obsessions, fixations and desires of the beach, no doubt exacerbated by the sultry weather and a surfeit of fresh air, are all-consuming. Sporting passions, communal passions, collective passions, passions *à trois*, passions *à deux*, no one is exempt. Take, for example, Fat Lugubrious Luis, disappointed college professor of something, summer seeker of the alternative life and also one of our neighbours. Every morning he puffingly pedals his long-suffering old bicycle through the rows of summer houses, gossiping, exchanging information, gathering, garnering. We watch his wobbling progress.

'It's not fair for the bike,' comments the Doctor.

'Where have you been, dear?' asks his sad unsmiling wife when he arrives home for his *cebiche* and siesta, his raw fish, lime and onion lunch and his rest.

'Cycling, dear,' replies Fat Lugubrious Luis. Or rather, recycling. It is his life source.

In the late afternoon he does the rounds again, just in case there have been any developments. This time he walks, puffing out his chest and raising his arms as he goes to show that he is fit and not fat.

'Here comes Water Melon Man,' whisper the mocking children peeping from between the lines of the multicoloured beach houses.

Not even the Doctor and La Señora are immune: they too are prey to the passions of the season. Predictably for the Doctor it is a straightforward matter of his horses and his porks: the farm is close by the straining beach house and he can readily escape to indulge his innocent pastime, or rather, immerse himself in his overriding obsession. And for the far-off races at El Hipódromo? A miniature hand-held radio has come into his possession, miracle of the modern world.

'I can hear barely,' he mutters, miracle of the modern world pressed to his ear. But it is enough. 'Once more fifth,' and he shrugs resignedly.

'Shessira?'

'No, Bertha.'

Ah, Big Bertha. With the lush glutes.

But La Señora, hot-blooded and artistic, is seized by other compulsions. Unfortunately, they lead to the regrettable and semi-scandalous episode of The Tortured Nude. The beginning is innocent enough. To the astonishment of all, our bank manager coyly announces his intention to get married. Not that anyone goes so far as to suggest that it is a belated attempt to prove the possession of at least some elements of humanity. Touched to tears by the romantically joyous news, soft-hearted La Señora unhesitatingly decides to present the betrothed, not-so-young couple with a gift of her very own making, a finely painted portrait. Nothing could be more appropriate to the occasion than her choice of subject: a reclining nude of heroic proportions. Doubly appropriate, seeing that our bank loan for the Clinic is of similar dimensions. For my part, I hope that the granite-hearted banker will be so overwhelmed by the naked gift that conceivably our rate of interest, per anum, of course, may be adjusted from the currently indigestible high teens into single figures. Merely a benign form of the ancient and time-honoured custom of 'payment in nature'.

Unsullied by such mercenary thoughts, La Señora loses no time in transferring her glowing feelings to the easel. Those who give quickly give twice. Removed from her Lima atelier, what better studio for the artist than the worn grass patch in front of the beach house? The brushes are wielded with a will and in no time at all, there is the banker's nude, reclining in the garden, exposed to the prurient public gaze. Herein lies the problem. Every beach-bound stroller stops to observe the art-full work on display, to admire, discuss, suggest and salivate.

The advice is unceasing, never mind the absence of artistic knowledge or talent. This is about female anatomy, everyone is an expert, the deprived husbands excelling. Appraising eyes inspect the embarrassed nude. Hmmmm, say the critics, maybe the thighs could be a little more inviting, perhaps the breasts are a touch too pendulous, too peachy; *las nalgas*, those generous buttocks, a fraction too majestic. Oxymorons abound.

Emanating from the family, such observations receive cursory dismissal.

'Please do not direct my paint,' says the artist. 'This is my personality on the canvas.'

That is the end of the matter. But for guests, La Señora is graciously accommodating, the perfect hostess. The artist listens attentively and makes the necessary adjustments. A small glass is shared with the visitors and the day progresses. More advice, more adjustments. Up go the breasts, down go the buttocks, in comes the stomach, out go the thighs. More delicate strokes on the inside leg, the hint of a caress just there, highlight this, emphasize that. A touch more luxuriant there. Another small glass is poured and shared.

At nightfall, The Tortured Nude is brought inside and mercifully laid to rest, the dust sheet is adjusted, as over a canary's cage. Tomorrow is another day, the wedding still a fortnight distant. Tiring work it is, in out, up down, constantly changing shape. Not just that. The Tortured Nude changes colour too. Sometimes pale and interesting, un-sunned, untouched by the light of day; sometimes nipple pink, rosily verging on the over-cooked. Other days bright red, gaudy with embarrassment no doubt. Green, purple, orange, every imaginable shade, like a demented rainbow. It all depends who passes, what advice is proferred. Unsurprisingly her expression becomes careworn, no longer the starry-eyed young bride, full of false hope. More the long-suffering wife. Thin lips, hollow cheeks, accusing eyes.

'*¡Cara seria, culo alegre!*' opines the Doctor professionally as he returns from a day with his horses and porks. He wisely makes a rapid escape and there is no time for a translation. We forgive La Señora any momentary lapses in concentration and application. Demanding work it is.

The great day dawns and The Tortured Nude is framed for posterity. One buttock pert and retroussé, the other inclined to flaccidity, revealing the effects of gravity; one breast appetizingly succulent, the other, well, less welcoming. One thigh Rubenesque, the other, well, not so comfortably accommodating. Something for all tastes. Double value in my humble judgement, two for the price of one.

The presentation is made, with apprehensive charm.

'Nice frame,' sniffs the banker, like a man from Sotheby's, oblivious to the suffering endured by The Tortured Nude, and the artist. Shortly afterwards our interest rate climbs another two points. Philistine. Some people have no artistic appreciation. Next time we will give him what he deserves: a 'thin-flanked woman, as white and as stale as a bone'. But who knows how high the interest might have gone without the influence of the nice frame enveloping The Tortured Nude? Then again . . .

'These Bank people put me nervous,' La Señora tells us. 'But you will see. I can put them nervous back.'

Sure enough, and by propitious way of consolation, La Señora is bestowed at this time with a surprise invitation to participate in forthcoming World Ice Sculpture Championships to be held in Sweden. The precise source of the honour remains unknown. The long reach of the artistic tendrils? Friends of friends? A Victorian tea-room conversation finally bearing fruit? Who you know, not what? A chronic dearth of Peruvian ice chippers? A little blurring of exactitude is sometimes for the best. It is a far cry from the baking beaches and bikinis of Cañete, but it more than suffices to restore La

112

Señora's artistic spirit. The invitation is accepted with alacrity; the necessary arrangements are set in hand.

'I will be fifteen days frozen, but I am going,' is La Señora's declaration. Then she reminds us: 'From fantasies come beautiful realities.'

Ah! The dreamers of the day who make their dreams come true.

Nearer to home a cloud passes over the sunlit sands. The brash banker, newly wed, assures us that business is booming. 'Your Clinic is a golden mine,' he declares.

For him, perhaps. Mr President of Peru tells us there is a world recession. That's not the message from Mr Dow Jones in New York. The problem appears to be a little more local. The Peruvian depression is deep and seemingly endless; businesses fold, jobs are lost, unemployment rises (although not according to the official statistics), nothing sells, hard times indeed. Rich pickings for the vultures. Whatever, our beautiful Clinic and La Señora's grand humanitarian strategy deserve better than this, her cherished vision of opening those charitable medical centres for impoverished Peruvians in areas of need, to be funded by the proceeds from The Ladies' Healthcare Clinic in Lima. Sites are being identified, plans made, the way paved. Except that at this moment, as hard as we may try, the Bank is laying claim to all the profits and there is not a solo centimo to spare. We feel like treadwheel hamsters, round and round to nowhere. If it wasn't the moment for *La Capea*, Carnival, *El Festival de Taurino* and *La Pamplonada* we might even be joining the Peruvian economy and suffering a mild case of depression ourselves. Happily, the distant Clinic has been entrusted to the safest hands available and here in Cañete diversions and entertainments are imminent.

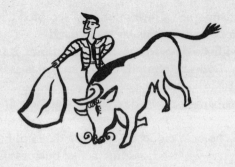

11

La Capea

It so happens that near our beach in Cañete is an old bullring, a surviving relic from the big hacienda that farmed these parts in the era, halcyon for some, prior to the infamous and disastrous 'agrarian reform' instituted in the early seventies by embittered General Juan Velasco's military junta. In those days La Señora's family also had a grand hacienda, hectares and countless hectares of rolling grassland 12,000 feet up on the Puno plateau on the shores of Lake Titicaca. Now, she tells us, the grand house is practically in ruins, the grazing mismanaged or abandoned.

'Oh, it was so large that you could never see the end of the edge,' explains La Señora. 'We lived there, all of us. It was our home. But then we had to leave. Everything.'

As for the bullring at Cañete, the proximity of such a treasure is too much for the Doctor, matador manqué. Every year in early February he is the instigator of *La Capea*. An afternoon of mini-bullfights with mini-bulls, just for fun. No killing, no blood. Well, not normally. And of course the gringo is invited. How very kind. To take part. Really? Of course! Just for fun.

So I take part. I don't really feel brave enough for such an event, except that I haven't the courage to decline. It would be easier to be an anonymous spectator, giving advice and passing judgement, as spectators do. But the moment is inopportune for such shaming revelations. As is often the case, the solution lies in a good lunch. Thereafter I feel much better and almost equal to the task ahead.

My participation in the parade of the toreadors is uneventful. We pay the customary respects to the judges, the participants thin out and take cover behind the boards and there we are, the moment of truth. Another glass of wine would be helpful at this point, but there is not a waiter to be seen. It's always the way. Just the Doctor and me in the dusty ring. The sun is scorching down on us like a laser, expectant vultures are circling lazily high overhead. Maybe I could just slip out and get a glass of water? Maybe not. No time for that, for out of the darkness of the tunnel here comes the pounding bull, nostrils belching steam, eyes flashing, tail lashing angrily.

¡U-ay! ¡Caramba! Where did they find such an animal? I have taken the wise precaution of removing my glasses for the occasion, but through the mist I myopically adjudge that this blurred beast must be all of 800 furious kilograms, packed with aggressive muscle and ferocious sinew. *Caramba* again! Now fire is coming out of its slobbering ugly mouth and just look at those horns! Must be almost two metres between the vicious tips. I really could use that glass of wine, water, anything. It's amazing how thirsty I feel watching this bull thundering towards us.

Happily, the Doctor takes first turn. He is quite neat with the *capote*, the scarlet cape; nice little pass, turns with a flourish. ¡Olé! My go. Without making a thing about it, I really think it wouldn't have been too much to ask for a waiter to have been on hand at this moment. Instead, all I have in hand is the *capote*.

Just that between me and a lingering, agonizing death. Actually, when I look at the bull again, and I am doing so frequently in these moments, I realize that death would be instantaneous. The bull is sizing me up, pawing the ground impatiently, half the length of a cricket pitch from where I am transfixed. The thought of cricket strengthens my resolve. I think of Queen and Country, this is what it was like in the days of Empire against the foreign foe. The Thin Red Line, Johnny Foreigner, all that sort of thing. 'Batting for the Empire, batting for the Raj, batting for the honour of the Crown.'

'Aheeee! Ahaaaa!' I cry provocatively at my gigantic tormentor, echoing the professionals calling to the bull in Plaza de Acho. 'Ahaaaa! Aheeee!' I shout again. Then, just like the real matadors, I throw my head back contemptuously to indicate to the bull that I am ready, I have no fear, come and get me if you dare. Nothing happens. Just my misfortune to get a deaf bull. The silence in the packed spectator stands is oppressive. What next? Who am I to know? The *capote* is heavier than I thought, my arms are beginning to ache.

Wayheyaeee! The bull is on the move, rapidly and in my direction. Decision time. I am suddenly uncertain whether to move the cape or my feet to deceive the advancing beast. And anyway, what if the bull doesn't know the rules and follows my feet when he should be following the cape? I really could have done with a little more training and advice. No time to consult the Doctor, who in any case appears to have disappeared. By chance, the sweaty beast trundles past sportingly and I relax and think about waving to the fans. Good bull! Well played! A near miss, but nicely executed. By the bull, that is.

This is easy. With a twirl of my *capote* I turn to face the jolly bull, ready for more. But behind my back the deceitful animal has been quicker. Not so sporting after all. There it is, on me, smelly thing, pushing and shoving, quite unnecessarily and unpleasantly. This is undignified, not the way it is supposed to be and, moreover, I am losing ground. Still no sign of the Doctor. Surely this should be his turn? Now that the bull is closer, well, right on top of me in fact, I see that it is smaller and younger than at first I thought. Poor little creature. Quite strong though, and I am still losing ground. Things are beginning to get out of hand but I think I see a way out of my predicament. Yes! It's not a classic move, but I drop the heavy *capote* over the bull's head. This has two positive effects, not only blindfolding the beast but also relieving my aching arms. Obvious really and I can't think why the regular matadors haven't perfected this move for themselves. I make a mental note that if and when I extricate myself alive from my current precarious situation I should take out a patent on my invention.

Next, by instinct, I take the bull by the horns. Not so original but even so it's not in the book and once again I catch him by surprise. After a moment or two of sharp wrestling I manage to spin my confused adversary directly away from me. Then I give him a brisk whack and off he trots, more or less obediently. But I know my advantage will be short-lived. Already the bull is tossing his head to dislodge the cape, then he will be back at me, eager to level the score. So I cut and run. I have done my bit and I am off. Bring on the Doctor, he's played before. My twinkling toes carry me to the barrier in a flash, my training regime after the Morro Solar robbery paying dividends in an unexpected direction. Up and over the railing and I am safe, full of bravado and hot air, pulse pounding. The view is better from here and I am forced to agree with the critics. Bullfighting is cruel: cruel for the matadors.

Now I see the Doctor down in the ring. He is beckoning. Forever beckoning. Does he want me to do a lap of honour? No. He has a theory that if two bullfighters stand shoulder to shoulder and confront the charging animal then the bull will pass harmlessly between them as they shimmy to the side. I indicate unequivocally that he will have to find another dummy to prove his theory. I am not one to hog the limelight and anyway, there is no way I am leaving the security of the stands. There is a limit to the things a man can be expected to do in a single afternoon, especially after such a good lunch. As for the Doctor's theory, it will probably remain just that until the end of time. Can't he see that these stupid bulls just haven't read the rules?

After my triumph I am ready to give a press conference, as they do in the Sheraton and Country Club hotels after *las corridas de toros* in Lima, saying how it was for me, what I thought of the bull (not a lot), the weather and the crowd. What I had for lunch, who I might have for dinner. All those kind of important things. But there are no press present, not even a photographer. Nevertheless, the toreros discuss the events of the afternoon excitedly and at length, this being an indispensable part of the sport.

'*El gringo es muy valiente,*' I hear them say. 'The gringo is very brave.'

I lower my head modestly. I sense that La Señora momentarily sees me in a new, more radiant light. Not merely as someone to carry the shopping.

'Now you can rich your book and grow your story,' she tells me with maternal pride.

I agree. I can retire with honour now. It will just be a slim volume. *Memoirs of a Bullfighting Man*. Then the dream is shattered.

'*No,*' says an authoritative voice, '*El gringo es inconsciente.*'

Yes, 'unknowing' is precisely the word. It is true. Completely unknowing, that's me. And I have no immediate plans for abandoning the stands to find out more. I have learnt quite enough to last a lifetime.

The following morning I have a slight headache. Just a normal hazard of the job. One of the fearsome bull's horns must have grazed my head during a daring reverse pass, with twirl and feint. We matadors have to expect the odd knock or two. Nothing that a glass or so of wine won't cure.

A complex dialogue between life and death indeed.

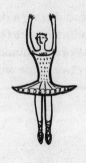

12

Carnival

After the raw drama and high tension of *La Capea*, the advent of Carnival comes as a welcome relief. In Lima the event is an excuse for the youth of the city to throw water over fellow citizens going about their lawful occasions; only spoilsports (like me) fail to appreciate just what a hilarious activity this is. On the beach at Cañete the preoccupation of the season is less active and more introspective. What to wear for the big parade? That is the question.

La Señora, our artistic director, regales us with tales of successes in years gone past, when armies of seamstresses with nimble fingers and broad behinds had created gorgeous butterflies, exotic birds, yodelling sea anemones and a whole medley of similar fantasies to delight the eye and win the heart of the judges. Accordingly, as the great day approaches I maintain my composure and await orders, like a highly trained greyhound in the starting trap, secure in the knowledge that a winning formula is at the very moment being polished and perfected.

'I see you are keeping stiff the lip,' observes Medical Student One, shrewdly.

I nod easily and confidently. After what I had been through in *La Capea* this little show was going to be a picnic. I watch and wait without comment as La Señora busily and lengthily attends numerous late-evening planning meetings with the ladies of the beach.

The great day dawns. Still no orders from High Command. Now I feel like a paratrooper, a coiled spring of steel poised in the open door at 10,000 feet, coolly waiting for the green light. Still nothing. I take some sun on the seashore, trying to concentrate on a worn copy of the Royal Horticultural Society *Journal* lent to me by La Señora. At teatime, I saunter back to the beach house. There is La Señora under the shade of the big umbrella, restorative, health-giving cucumber slices resting disconcertingly in each eye like two monocles from the local joke-store.

'So,' I say brightly, 'what's it to be then?' Even greyhounds and paratroopers have their limits.

'*¿Qué?*' The cucumber slices stare at me interrogatively. 'What?'

'Giraffes? Tigers on stilts? Humming birds? Illuminated snails? Articulated electric eels? Fluorescent slugs? Lizards?' I run out of inspiration.

'Nothing.'

'Nothing?' Why is it that I am always having this kind of non-conversation?

'Nothing. We are not taking part this year. I am upset.'

I can't believe it. La Señora is 'upset'. Well, now I am upset too. The lollipop snatched from my lips and dashed to the ground. Life can be so cruel. But I know better than to ask questions. When High Command has spoken, well, that's it. Finished. Game over. 'Never explain, never complain', that's what I was taught. Hands in pockets, kicking a stone along the path, I slouch back to my lent copy of the Horticultural *Journal*.

But I just can't seem to get into it. I am only grateful that Medical Student One doesn't pass by with any more shrewd observations.

Then, suddenly, all change!

'All right then,' says High Command decisively, leaping from her sunbed with the cucumbers jumping from her eyes. 'If that's what you want, we'll do it!'

By jingo! This is it! Green light on, action stations! The orders come thick and fast now.

'Take your clothes off!'

'*¿Perdón?*' It's one thing for greyhounds, but for paratroopers? Well . . .

High Command disappears into the beach house loft. Amazing, what a treasure trove, a regular Pandora's Box! I can go as Mickey Mouse, Moby Dick, Flash Gordon, The Man in the Moon, Popeye, Roger the Lodger, anything. I don't mind really, I just want to be in the parade. But Popeye would be fun . . .

'Alicia Alonso.'

'*¿Perdón?*'

'You are going as the celebrated ballerina. Are you in the process of disassembly? No? Not yet? TAKE YOUR CLOTHES OFF!'

Well, as dresses go, I suppose it isn't bad. Sort of orange, lots of frills and a daring neckline, not that I am too concerned about that.

'You don't need a wig.'

'*¿Per—?*' Oh, never mind. I'll take it as a compliment.

'And hurry up and get undressed. We haven't got much time.'

The Doctor agrees to accompany me, on humanitarian grounds. He has a flat cap handy and a black polo neck sweater and decides to be music-man Chichi Peralta. The make-up department do the rest. Not bad at all. High Command tosses some glitter-dust over me and we, Chichi and me, that is, make our way to the assembly point. I mingle with the other artistes, and catch one or two admiring glances coming in my direction. Even envious, I imagine. I flutter my eyelashes, breathing in deeply and pushing out my ballooning chest. Fancy going through life with these things in front of you. High Command reappears.

'You're next.'

'¿*Per*—?' When I am nervous I sometimes repeat myself.

'That's your music now. On you go.'

'Where's Chichi? Where's the parade?'

'There isn't any parade. It's individual acts.'

'Individual acts!' I don't mean to sound hysterical, but I am and I do.

High Command gives me an enormous shove. This is worse than *La Capea*. That bull was more gentle and caring than La Señora. I don't even have a *capote* to drop over her head. As I freefall from 10,000 feet into the glare of the footlights I feel certain La Señora has had military training. She was a Sergeant Major, Special Forces. Now I am sure of it. And another thing, I need to have a quiet word with the Doctor. He's becoming as elusive as a bar of soap in the shower. I blink and presto! He's gone! A bottled genie in reverse. It's too much.

But there is no time to think about all that now. I have reached the dropping zone. A thousand pairs of eyes are on me. I never realized it was going to be like this. Nothing, nothing prepared me for this. That's what the veterans always say. The audience is seated expectantly at various tables, the nice compère has announced Alicia Alonso and my ballet music is playing.

I panic. I want out. Now! The make-up department have removed my glasses and what with the spotlights and footlights and headlights and sidelights I am confused. Like a startled rabbit I scuttle across the arena, seeking the exit, my feet moving by remote control in time with the music. Furious applause. I stop, paralysed with stage fright, pirouetting slowly. The audience is ecstatic. My feet move off again, those twinkling toes.

'Bravo! Bravo!' cry the fans. 'Encore!'

I get the message. 'The roar of the grease paint, the smell of the crowd.' Another pirouette, *en point*, and there I go again. My word, fame at last! I go for a huge Nureyev leap and hang tantalizingly in the air, lingering in space, defying gravity. The noise is deafening. Right, get out while I'm ahead! I make another attempt to find the exit, only to find my way barred by the judges' table. Bad luck, but thinking quickly I turn the setback to advantage and kiss all three of the male adjudicators. Overconfident, I essay a curtsey in front of the one female member of the panel and have the misfortune to slip. Whoops! Definitely time to leave. This time Lady Fortune is with me and with the applause ringing in my ears I lift my skirts, or rather, my tulle tutu, and hurtle through a narrow gap between the packed tables. Straight into the arms of a waiter. This is better than *La Capea* after all. A nice glass of white wine, chilled too.

High Command is waiting for me. I give a nonchalant smile and wait for the Medal of Honour to be pinned to my amply inflated bosom. But the balloons never burst.

'Get that make-up off, get disassembled,' she snaps. 'What do you want people to take you for?'

'You mean . . . ?'

'Exactly.'

My goodness, a member of the pink sock brigade! We don't want that.

Then I spot the Doctor.

'Sorry,' he tells me. 'By the time we arrived they already had another Chichi Peralta.'

A little later in the evening I am called forward to receive a handsome prize from the judges. For valour and talent or out of compassion? The gringo will never know. But he can guess.

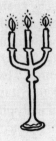

13

Two Funerals and Some Weddings

Yet another Clinic finance planning meeting slides incon-
clusively into desultory oblivion. We are seated round the
conference table in the auditorium and as usual we are in
stockinged feet in deference to the Scandinavian floorboards.
The big TV screen gazes down on proceedings blankly; no
World Cup football today, not even a closed circuit nicely executed buttock tuck courtesy of Dr Cleeber's deftly wielded
scalpel.

On one side of the auditorium-cum-gymnasium are three
lofty, ecclesiastically pointed windows looking out on our
ever-curious neighbours; the inner wall of the room is given
over to an immense mirror in the narcissistic manner of the day
so that the exercising ladies may admire whatever there is to
be admired. For finance meetings the effect is less pleasing and
less positive, as all our contentious deliberations are reflected
and mimicked in duplicate, such as ill-received entreaties to

125

dispose of some of our assets, spare holdings of land and the odd vehicle or two, for example, followed by violent reactions and virulent expostulations from predictable quarters.

Glass double-doors in the far corner of the room lead on to an internal patio, open to the sky two floors above. Here there are plans, yet to be realized, to install a whimsical water feature whereby a calming cascade will splash sonorously into a blue-tiled pool. My suggestion to decorate the area additionally with a selection of exotically foliaged tropical ferns and to add a few fish has not met with favour, presumably on health and snake grounds, so that all that is lacking is the perpetual motion circulating water-pump. Peruvian procurement is proving to be a greater problem than anticipated and to date a succession of suavely erudite engineers more accustomed to installing vast hydroelectric turbines in the mountains have visited, discussed, taken lunch, deliberated and finally declared the challenge to be beyond their oily capacities. Secretly I am quite relieved as I pessimistically sense the project has potential for flooding on a Noachian or even Manolian scale, yet again to the detriment of the warp-prone flooring.

Thus it is that for the time being our fractious finance meetings are conducted without the benefit of rhapsodic aquatic accompaniment and as usual the convenient concluding consensus is that we are doing well but not quite well enough. Like the blank TV screen, the equally empty bookshelves of the yet-to-be-acquired medical library on the balcony encircling the upper reaches of the auditorium survey the scene in solemn and silent condemnation.

The Doctor consults his watch meaningfully, considers the information thus imparted and escapes on urgent business. Señorita Hilda sighs profoundly, as might an expiring whale, and with countenance grave sets about collecting the cheerless cups and saucers whilst Ernestina absent-mindedly puts the budget projections back in the folder for another day, her thoughts turning to the jam whirligig she has secreted in the bottom drawer of her desk.

'I think you are a wedding person,' declares La Señora, apropos of nothing and by way of moving our lives forward on to more agreeable matters. 'You are not for funerals.'

I am equally ready to forget the finances and, on balance, I hope that she is right. Not that you always get the choice. Moreover, given the size of La Señora's extended family it is inevitable that during our preoccupation with the Clinic and Cañete, Cañete and the Clinic, there should be happenings.

The first was a distant funeral, away from Lima. It is easy to be brave at distant funerals. No tears. The discussion is detached, the details impersonal.

'They were good friends on the gate between the gardens,' explains La Señora. 'She lost her friend over the garden wall.' That's it, nothing else.

Funerals should get easier with practice. Instead, they become harder with time. Until, that is, effortlessly it becomes your turn. When the years are with you, a funeral is an irrelevance, something that happens to other people. When the years are against you, you feel the chill wind and you look over your shoulder. Who's next? You cheat a little, and think of other things to maintain composure when the coffin passes. Dying must be like staying in bed on a cold morning. For ever.

Our second funeral is in Lima. It is close. Too close. Uncle Parcemon of Miraflores, for it is he, now deceased, was my friend. Long retired and frequent casual caller at the Clinic, Señor Parcemon was everybody's friend, everybody's uncle. I learnt to recognize his footfall on the stairs to my office as, several times a week, he would drop by to see how things were in England, how was the King nowadays? And Mr Churchill? He is also well? Then we might take a turn round the potted plants and gently venture into Peruvian politics over the petunias.

Very early on the morning of his departure, the new day still dark and chill, Uncle Parcemon sends word to me in the Clinic that he is packing his bags in readiness to leave for the great hereafter. No footfalls on the stairs, instead a mosquito wakes me on the fourth floor in the small hours to pass the tidings but I fail to read the signal and try to kill the messenger. Pswish, pswish, round the room with the spray can. Meanwhile, over the invisible border into San Isidro, the Doctor is similarly awakened in Casa Bonomini by an uninvited bug knocking and tapping in his bedside lamp. He too fails to read the message. Every time he puts the lamp on to catch the rattling messenger, it disappears, while La Señora tosses and turns so much that the bed has to be remade.

'Sorry,' Uncle Parcemon is saying, 'but I'm on my way; I'm tired now. I have lived the earthly journey and I have to go. The complications and disappointments in my life have multiplied beyond my capacity to bear them.'

But it is not until the telephone rings at breakfast-time that we comprehend the news and understand. It was a life that had become too 'heavy with existence'.

'We must always be ready,' reflects the Doctor. 'Ready with our luggage. You can prepare for the next life but it can be at any time.'

Waiting for the funeral service, panacea for the living, we tell the story of the rattling bug and the whining mosquito to Parcemon's neighbour.

'*¿Casualidad? ¿Coincidencia? ¿Intencionalidad?*' she asks meaningfully in that soft voice of hers.

Chance, coincidence, or something more? We nod knowingly, softly and equally meaningfully. The twenty-first century will surely open the doors of the extrasensory, the telepathic, the Fourth Dimension. Just head to head, or better still, heart to heart. Farewell to modems, blighted e-mail, all those telephone bills.

'That lady is a mystic,' we declare to one another after the Requiem Mass. And we recall how she extinguishes the long candles in her house with a conical snuffer, so that the warm wishes and gentle spirits are contained and do not blow away and escape on the faint swirls of drifting smoke. But Dr Hermogenes is unconvinced.

'Just dumb,' he declares, uncharacteristically forthright.

The Catholic funeral rites completed, the transient mourners take their impatient leave, anxious to rejoin the living, and the lonely widow, once an enchanted bride, more recently my friend's wife, is left to clear the clutter and to pack Uncle Parcemon's life, now also departed, into boxes. 'Now I must pick up the pieces of the rest of my life,' she tells herself bravely in the echoingly empty solitude of the deserted house. 'But in truth my soul will forever dance the slow waltz of sadness and my hidden grief will never end. Look, my dearest husband, my dearest heart, wherever you may be, the moon is among my tears and you may see them in the midnight sky, lonely, shining and waiting for you.'

The family wedding is wedding number five for Grandfather Ulises. He beams his way benignly and confidently through the ceremony, not a trace of nerves. Clear proof that for weddings, unlike funerals, practice makes perfect. But it is La Señora's turn to be sceptical.

'Don't forget that he is taking pills for the brain,' she says cryptically. 'And others,' she adds, mysteriously. 'At this moment he has the emotion of going to a party that will never end. He doesn't want to know that someone has set the clock to close the door.'

No, Ulises definitely doesn't want to think about anything

like that. He knows now that all his marriages are triumphs of hope over experience but after the collapse of his lyrical dreams in his first union, he subscribes to the school of thought that with matrimony you just have to keep plugging away in the belief that you may strike lucky in the end. That is, unless the money runs out first. And anyway, at the age of twenty-one the first marriage is for ever, which is a very long time. Now he is past the age of seventy the chances are that he won't have to keep things going for quite so long, thereby shortening the odds against failure, or rather, improving the possibility of success. However, the Doctor is less sanguine.

'Don't forget that love can drag you further than dynamite can blow you,' he reminds us pointedly. 'You would imagine that at his age Ulises should be able to think further than the bedroom,' he reflects. Then he reflects some more. 'No. Perhaps I am momentarily mistaken. Possibly it is because of his age that his vision is limited. But whatever the cause, now he must steer his lonely course. He is like a ship without the Captain on the bridge, heading implacably for the inevitable rocks of regret.'

Goodness gracious, this is strong stuff. Maybe the Doctor is right. Except I have a feeling, only sneaking, of course, that when the shipwreck comes, Ulises will lie there on the shore, damp and dented. And with a contented smile on his lips, insulated against the bitterness of life, exhausted and penniless though he may be, he will say to himself: 'My word, that was marvellous! Absolutely marvellous. Now I can die in peace.' Many are the conventions of life, but happily this diverse world of incomprehensible complexity is inhabited by just a sprinkling of the unconventional. Such a one is Grandfather Ulises.

But what of the bride? Also past the age of blushing, Luzmila too is wearing a quiet smile to complement her sensible suit and floral bonnet. But hers is a smile of triumph.

'Do tell us the secret of your success,' beg her disappointed friends with bright eyes and bitter envy in their hearts. And the enigmatic bride smiles demurely, knowing that those who have to ask the question will not understand the answer.

'Oh, it's easy,' she explains ingenuously. 'Always with your mouth you should just blow flowers to your man. Put trust in the perfume of the flowers and Christian Dior. You must proud him a little and never leave him without the taste of honey. And always hold his hand and tight the fingers very much. Finally, should there ever be an upset, turn your face and don't put any more fire on the fire.'

Sound advice indeed, although perhaps she is overlooking the possibility that 'now the bride is in the bed, all the promises are dead'. Let battle commence.

La Señora has solidly settled opinions on the subject of matrimony.

'I have the experience. I do not want to say that I am an excellent person, just a normal person, but I was grown to be a good wife. That was good lessoning for me, it made everything clear and bright. I learnt very deeply, then my mother put me to the church. It was my turn to get married so I did that. My mother said you marry this person, he is a doctor and you get sick all the time. My mother was very known. She was such a happy person. She could move the world with her happiness. She wanted me to be a serious woman, she was celebrating getting rid of me. Two thousand people came to my wedding, with lots of food and drinks. That is how it was in Peru in those days. Five months later I was pregnant and so I became a serious woman.' La Señora pauses and, yes, the hush is expectant.

'Marriage is like two columns, you must let the air pass through it. Or more exactly, you must "let the winds of the heavens dance between you". You may think that marriage is a natural occurrence. Not entirely, only some aspects of the situation. Much better if you accept now that although you will probably marry, overall and in general it is an unnatural condition. You need someone to fight the life with you, not someone you have to carry. Then you have the best jewel in your life. The marriage should balance: she provides the spoon, he provides the lamp. Some of these girls do not even bring a bra and knickers to the altar. When I married I had the diamonds on the neck and two feather blankets but not one penny. No underwear, just the mink coat. We arrived at our house in the night so we knew no one in the morning. We had to ring the bells and say please help us. Of course you must marry for love, but it is helpful if you can love where money is. And if you are a man, never make the mistake of trying to understand the finer thoughts of a woman. Just accept that you will never understand and know that women come from another planet more advanced than yours. If you doubt my words, try in vain to find in a man those magical qualities of inner grace, of silent elegance and calm modesty possessed by so many women. From my deep inside, this is what I think. I am speaking from my very deep, everything I say is from the deep of my heart and this is what you must know. Oh yes. One thing more. Again, if you are a man you may admire the form and beauty of a woman. But always check the feet. Only consider marriage to a woman with active feet.'

And to *las señoritas*, the young brides of tomorrow, she is equally outspoken.

'Let me talk to you something. Carefully listen. I am a primitive woman. I learn from what I see around. I am a good student, but I am a better teacher. I have the power of knowledgement in my hands and in my fingers. When you are young, you are in the age of discovery. You may seek advice but in the finality always listen to your inner voice. If you find a good man that you love you may go ahead, accept him and marry him even if he doesn't have shoes for the wedding. He will be happy, sometimes we have to do a little step in our lives to help another one. Look at the horizon and always be thinking, what can I do here for helping? It is your responsibility to put sparkling dust into your marriage. The essence of life is not the sex. It is the love. That is the thing that moves the world. And the money, of course. In your life there will come just one big wave. Be sure to hold on to your wave. Or it will pass like a feather in the wind. Remember that love never changes. People change, love is constant. And also remember that you can control a man's temper through his stomach. If you feed him too much meat he will be difficult in the night. If you feed him fish then he will be satisfactory. But if he starts acting strange, then you must get rid of him.'

'*Querida Tía*, dear Aunt Coraima, what sort of strange?' enquire the libidinous young ladies, interest awakened.

'*Por ejemplo*, for example, if he starts wanting to wear your shoes in bed.' The young ladies are disappointed. 'I read that in a magazine,' concludes La Señora, by way of explanation. 'I am your older. Do your life this way. And remember, a lover is too expensive. Never marry for sex; when the *entusiasmo* passes everything is past. This is now the lesson's end; do these things and I will be very well pleased. For all this, patience a lot you need. And learn how to act like a rich without being. I am sorry to be so long in my speech but some things you have to explain vocally talking. Maybe this was a sermon for you. Hold my words very well strong. I believe that all sermons should go somewhere, although not necessarily very far. One day you will never forget me.'

She leaves us to think on that. And in different ways, we do, the wise amongst the listeners knowing that the precious bestowal of a woman's love is truly a divine gift from the gods in the heavens above, pure, abounding and without limits.

During the ceremony I notice that the Doctor is wearing red and white Mickey Mouse socks under his smart grey suit. He intercepts my eye and shrugs, sheepishly. Or mousily. Are the socks a commentary on the proceedings or has the laundry got confused in Casa Bonomini?

'This is just the suit I catch from the cupboard,' whispers Dr Hermogenes apologetically in my ear.

'Doctor,' I whisper back, giving a smile of encouragement, 'the suit is admirable.'

'Oh, *gracias*. Thank you,' he says with relief in his face.

It is not the moment for questions. I shall never know about the socks.

Family weddings are special occasions, but weddings in general are a regular feature of our social round. The offspring of long-standing friends and patients of the Clinic seem to be doing it all the time, accompanied by banqueting and dancing, and we receive a deluge of invitations. Surfeit or not, we do our best to attend, for the best of reasons. The clinical mind of Dr Hermogenes the philosopher is tireless in its musings and en route to yet another nuptial night out he shares with us his thoughts.

'Weddings,' he declares, choosing his words carefully, 'can catalyse christenings.' As ever, his professional logic is as impeccable as it is irrefutable, as befits one who is increasingly engaged in conducting deliveries for the second generation of the same family. But there is yet more gynaecological wisdom. 'And where there is one christening, others may follow.' No one speaks for quite some time.

Meanwhile, La Señora loses no opportunity to revive the fanciful legend of the visiting English Lord, garnishing the story with hints of riches, old money, many rolling acres and a stately home or two.

'I invent it, of course,' she breathes in my ear, 'but, well, now it is the truth.' Rumour, marinaded with time.

The scene at Cousin Jaime's wedding is typical. Waiting until La Señora is otherwise engaged, two painted ladies of a certain age approach our table. I see them coming and affect extreme myopia and total ignorance of Castellano, one being closer to the truth than the other.

'Does your friend dance?' they enquire of the Doctor, nodding in my direction.

¿A él, le gusta el azúcar? Does he take sugar? I gaze fixedly at my champagne glass, mesmerized by the bubbles.

'Ah! He used to,' sighs the Doctor heavily and then continues, selecting his similes carelessly, 'oh, how he danced, as light as a condor's feather and as graceful as a riverside willow in the evening breeze.'

I grip the stem of the glass, the bubbles are giving me trouble. The Doctor allows his eyes to mist a little. The ladies lean forward in suspense. He lowers his voice.

'That was before the accident.'

'The accident?' The ladies are startled but maintain unison.

'Yes, the accident.'

'The accident . . . ?'

'He was shot.'

'Shot!' The ladies leap an octave but the harmony is commendable. 'Where?'

'In the war.'

'Yes, yes, but where exactly?'

'In France, I believe.'

'No, no, the other whereabouts?'

'Oh, I see what you mean. In the leg, twice. Once low down, and then . . . ' the Doctor falters. Then he regains control and continues, confidentially. 'And once a little further up.'

'A little further up . . . ?' whisper the chorusing ladies repetitively, glancing furtively in my direction.

The Doctor nods, lost for words.

'Ah.' The downcast ladies take their leave.

There are some things money cannot buy.

When the approach is more direct, sometimes taken by surprise in the intimate seclusion of my fourth-floor office by a patient who has wandered up the stairs by premeditated mistake, then I am left to handle the situation less subtly without the aid of the Doctor.

'Come for dinner tonight.' A flicker of the eyes accompanies the proposal.

'No, thank you.' No blinking.

'Please yourself. But remember that we are only here once.' That flicker again.

'That's why I am not coming.' Then I spend the rest of the day seeking solace in the dead tree full of those hyperactive pigeons, thinking that maybe I should have blinked after all.

With true Peruvian hospitality, leavened with interest reserved for oddities, I am always kindly included in the many invitations, be they for engagements, weddings, christenings, anniversaries or, indeed, for any other sundry spontaneous supposition.

'The curiosity is here, like a peanut,' explains La Señora, 'these people they cannot love you less. They know yourself.'

'Oh.'

'They think you are beautiful.'

'Ah.'

'I have told them that you have a warm heart and that your help to us is unvaluable.'

We are usually an hour or so late: it is *la hora peruana*, an hour or so behind the clock. It is a matter of prestige. How could a busy *funcionario* possibly be *a la hora*, on time for anything? Moreover, in the rural world of *los Andinos* life is governed by the natural rhythms of the mountains: the sowing of the seed, the falling of the rains, the garnering of the harvest. Division of the day into hours, minutes and seconds is a contrived concept for the countryside. Sufficient to know that it is early in the day, around the middle of the day, or getting late. Well, that's the explanation – and the foundation of the belief that 'he who arrives *a la hora* is a clown'.

It is only visitors to Peru who have a problem with *la hora peruana*; they find it difficult to adjust, as though they had arrived in London in June and forgotten to change their watches to British Summer Time. For Peruvians the rules are simple, everyone is comfortably adjusted and in step. For example, a conversation might go like this:

Street vendor: 'Please collect the *juanes*, these delicious *tamales* of rice and meat wrapped in banana leaves, at noon tomorrow.'

Dr Hermogenes: 'I would like to know when is your noon. Is it one o'clock or two o'clock?'

Street vendor: 'It is twelve o'clock.'

Dr Hermogenes: 'Really? Then I will come sooner or later.'

Exactly. Easy.

Our punctuality problem is compounded by the fact that it is generally unwise to wear a conspicuous watch when travelling through the city of Lima and the environs. Like jewellery, watches tend to attract unwelcome envious attention.

'Never mind,' we agree cheerfully as we set off from Casa Bonomini, 'we can tell the time by the sun.'

'And with the sun in the clouds,' asks the Doctor empirically, 'how you do then?'

'By the stomach.'

'No,' says Medical Student One in that solemn way of his. 'We need a cat.' He reads a lot, does Medical Student One. 'If we had a cat we could tell the time.'

'What kind of cat? A Peruvian one for *la hora peruana*?'

Medical Student One ignores this frivolous interruption. 'You can tell the time by the dilation of its eyes.'

'You squeeze it by the neck?'

'If you like, but a cat's pupils dilate significantly depending on the amount of light available. You just need to calibrate the cat.'

'Calibrate the cat? Like a calibrated choirboy or a eunuch? Maybe after all we should bring a watch next time.'

'Yes,' agrees Medical Student One reluctantly, 'possibly it might be easier if we did happen to have a clock on hand.'

La hora Señora is not one but two hours behind the clock, which is pushing things a bit. For one of our many christening parties, memorable for the wrong reasons, we arrive the prescribed two hours late to find the church long deserted, with no way of knowing in which direction our hosts and their offspring, recently assisted into this world by no less a hand than that of Dr Hermogenes, had departed. Possibly word was left for us, but if so, now there is no trace of the messenger. In Peru, never ask anyone to pass a message; better to save your breath. It is a disappointment, a setback even. However, there are no heavy words on the subject, no recriminations. It seems that something similar may have happened before. Often. The Doctor calmly directs our car to a second party, yet another betrothal celebration of unrestrained optimism, which conveniently just happens to be taking place in the same vicinity and we receive the invariable warm welcome, regardless of the hour.

'At least we are late!' exclaims La Señora as we arrive at the revised venue, happily, forsaking clarity for honesty. We know what she means.

'Go ahead, go ahead,' say our new hosts, 'feel yourself at home.'

La Señora introduces me theatrically, avoiding my eye.

'The English Consultant,' she reveals with a flourish, as though I had sprung from a film première. Then she adds as an afterthought to fill the uncomprehending silence, 'We are proud of him very much.'

'Ah, he is an English toffee! Yes?' exclaim our surrogate hosts, happy with their sparkling wit.

'Yes, an old English toffee,' confirms La Señora, readily prolonging the sticky moment. 'He is very strict. Before he was a military man. It's a problem for him. At first he makes us cry a lot, but now we don't cry so much. He says that we lose a lot of time just talking and that punctuality is very important.'

Everyone surveys me doubtfully whilst I smile back weakly and try to look pleasant.

Another sticky moment but La Señora has yet to complete her vignette of the ogre.

'Now when he speaks to us all calmed down, we get nervous. I like him to shout, then I can shout back.'

Then, on conclusion of the courtesies, my opinion is sought on the topics of the day, mainly political. In turn, I seek La Señora's advice.

'I am just a visitor in your country. I don't have the right to—'

'That is a big lie,' she retorts. 'The people want to hear what the foreigners think. You are the only English here; they are all turning to you. You are the one looking through the window. You must say what you see.' Then it is her turn to gaze at me doubtfully. 'Or else they might think that perhaps you are thinking and seeing nothing. Are you the red light or the green light? Or just the yellow light? Or perhaps you are a floating cloud? Nice to meet you, Mr Cloud!'

If only La Señora knew. However, I must do my best. My interlocutor opens the bowling with a full toss from the pavilion end.

'Señor, do you consider it a surprise that the President is standing for a third term of office when the constitutional rules specifically state that two terms is the maximum permissible?'

'Er, yes, I think "surprised" is exactly the right word.'

'Señor, do you also agree it is surprising that the majestic moonscape adjacent to the Pan Americana Sur, the motorway, can be defiled by mindless political graffiti comprising giant slogans on every second mountainside?'

I gain confidence. These questions are just looseners. 'I think it is diabolical.'

'Diabolical?'

I lose confidence. 'Er, rather surprising.'

'Ah, yes, rather surprising. And do you also agree, señor,

that it is surprising that nothing is done about the *invasores* who, in a sinister breakdown of law and order, descend from the hills in their thousands and squat on privately owned prime agricultural land?'

Careful now. I need to have a further audience with La Señora. Urgently.

'Señor, whilst you are thinking about that, is it true that in Europe they believe that here in Peru we still wear feathers?'

'Feathers? Well, er, you know, in England a lot of people still wear feathers in their caps, I mean hats. At Ascot and that sort of thing.'

'I see.' The unseeing eyes are unwavering. 'Señor, before you leave us, would you agree that Peru is not Third World, it is a developing country, in fact it is a project for a country not yet a country, and that it could be said that Third World is a state of mind, a psychological sickness, which unfortunately one does encounter from time to time?'

'Er, could you repeat the question please?' Or was it a statement?

'Señor, and might you not agree that here in Peru we suffer the morally handicapped in high places and that as a result of this intrinsic lack of moral values there is a thread of dishonesty running through all aspects of life, political, commercial and domestic?'

This is getting worse. But yes, now that you mention it, where is Truth? It has indeed stumbled in the street. I pause and my eyes roll as I look for the exit. Why do I spend so much of my life looking for the exit?

My interlocutor edges closer. 'Maybe you would wish to say it is a river of dishonesty?' he murmurs in my ear.

'No, no! Not at all. Just a dribble, I mean hardly a trickle, not even a stream in the rainy season or rather, I mean the dry season.'

Yes, it's true, I am panicking, babbling like a brook. What

140

people don't hear, they make up. They will say that I said that 'in South America corruption is the indispensable grease of life's daily round'. But I didn't say that, someone else did. I only thought it, because my mind is fixated with the memory of a recently published world corruption league table, worst first. Peru languished somewhere in the upper echelons. It was not so much the predictable positioning that stuck in my mind. It was more the memory of Medical Student One poring over the survey with furrowed brow, offended by the findings.

'How come we came so low?' he puzzled. Then the light dawned. 'Ah yes, I see. Now I have it. Money changed hands.'

Yes, money is always changing hands, or hoping to. Long prior to my arrival in Lima the officials in the Town Hall had apparently engaged in spuriously delaying the required certification for opening the Clinic. Not by weeks, not by months, but for over a year. Finally we sat in the Mayor's office and declined to leave until we either had the vital document or an interview with the great man. We beat the system and left with our bit of paper, but even so, a few days later the mother of the principal official involved, a lady supposedly of some standing in the social carousel, called privately to seek the payment she felt was due to her son. She left unrewarded but also quite unabashed. What was that about a 'river of dishonesty' at all levels of society?

My interrogation continues.

'Well, you must surely agree that drunken drivers in general and drunken coach drivers in particular and lack of pollution control on old vehicles are real problems in Lima? And that the step from the donkey to the wheel, from four legs to the Ferrari, has been too short?'

'Yes, indeed. Definitely. And possibly.' Easy. Except for that bit about the donkey. How am I scoring? Badly. I seek refuge and consult La Señora.

'So, how should I have dealt with that question about dishonesty?'

'Just tell the truth. That will confuse everybody. I have learnt not even to trust my shadow in the mirror. Don't trust anyone here. I am telling that even when you look to the mirror do not believe that it is you. I can say to you that I put a mirror in my room but believe it or not it doesn't work. It is too high and I am too short.'

'And the Third World and the feathers?'

'For your years in Peru, don't you even think about the comparation,' says La Señora. 'We are proud of our feathers. Peru is the last country that nobody knows that is great. We are fresh Third World.'

'*Señor, por favor, una pregunta más.*' One more question? My *inquisidor* is back on my shoulder. 'How is it that you came to end here in Lima?'

Ah! Once again the statement within the question. Is this the end for me? I hadn't thought of it that way before. Maybe I should start, right now.

'Oh, I am just passing by, that's all.'

'I see. *Gracias, señor.*'

It's another 'I see' that doesn't see.

Sometimes I am mistakenly credited with medical knowledge.

'Doctor, *por favor*, how do you feel for this wedding cake?'

'Mmmmmm, delicious, thank you. What about you? Another slice, perhaps?'

'I am just wondering, in the abstract, if you would advise that we eat it every day?'

'Er . . . ' Something prompts me that this is not the moment for facetiousness. 'No, probably not. It's very good of course, but maybe just once or twice a week would be sufficient.' That's if there is sufficient. In the abstract, of course.

'Thank you. And now another consultation for free. How about the Coca-Cola? Every day, more or less?'

'Yes, that will be fine. You could always try pure water for a change.' Or a drop of whisky.

'Pure water? Thank you. Now could you inform me on Mr Shackspear? He was Chileno or Brasileño, *sí o no*?'

'It's quite possible. But many people say that he was English.'

'And you? How do you say?'

'Well, I've always rather understood that perhaps he was indeed English, and that at very least the renowned works were written by someone of a similar name.'

'Ah ha! I see! And your shirt, is that an example of British textiles?'

'Yes, actually. I hope you like it. British textiles, next to the skin, every day.'

'I see. Thank you, Doctor.'

There's none so blind as those that cannot see.

On other occasions the consultations are grammatical rather than literary-medicinal.

'Excuse me, sir, but please what does "creysi" mean?'

'Crazy?'

'*Sí*, creysi.'

'*Loco.*'

'*¿Loco?*'

'Yes, *loco*. For example, "I am crazy about you." Or even "I am crazy for you."'

'Ah! "I am creysi about you or even four you."'

'No. Not exactly.'

'Ah! "I am creysi four you or even about you, not exactly."'

'Yes! You've got it! Perfect.'

'*Gracias, señor.*' And my new-found friend trots off to put his new-found knowledge to good use. The best things in life are free, of course. Except that impromptu consultations without a price are sometimes exactly that. Worthless.

But more usually, and thankfully, I am the patient recipient of confidences and advice rather than the dispenser.

'If I were you,' I am told, in uncomfortably close confidence

143

and *a propósito de nada*, 'I would balance away from the carbo-hydrates and incline more to the drinking.'

This comes from rubicund Rudecindo, a man possessed of an enthusiastic complexion who seeks me out on every social occasion to remind me that before the disaster of agrarian reform the lands of his family hacienda stretched from *la costa* through *la sierra* to *la selva*. From the coast, across the mountains to the rainforests, connected by a privately owned railway. *¡Hombre!* Now, no doubt as a result of the disappoint-ment of the enforced loss, he spends his days following his own advice, inclining heavily towards the drinking and aban-doning the carbohydrates, so much so that after the first glass his mouth also inclines, causing his words to slip sideways from his lopsided lips, splashing their way wetly to the floor, often via my tie. For me there is no escape; Rudecindo is relent-less in his pursuit of a fresh pair of ears.

'From my profession I am a little retired just in this moment,' he confides, edging ever nearer and helping himself from a passing salver of *conchitas*. 'I am not using my mind too much in these moments.'

I watch spellbound as he misses his mouth and the scallop shoots over his shoulder to form an accusing puddle on the carpet. Rudecindo of the colourful complexion scarcely notices, his taste buds clutching at thin air.

'Politics?' he continues, seamlessly. 'In South America? Better to eat and drink. By the way, how many children do you have, roughly speaking?'

We can blame the non sequiturs on the slippery *conchita*.

On occasions we are the privileged recipients of more formal invitations.

'Look! Look!' exclaims La Señora excitedly, opening the crested envelope that has just been hand-delivered to the Clinic. 'Your Queen Elizabeth's mother has invited us to a party!'

On the appointed day we send crystal vases in advance containing rare orchids of exquisite fragility and that same evening duly proceed to the Embassy to celebrate the coming of age of the much-loved centenarian, singing 'Happy Birthday' in the hill-top garden of the Residence, high above the glittering lights of the district of Monterrico, Lima. Secretly we wish that we too will score a century with equal dignity and grace, whilst some of the guests wait impatiently for the arrival of Her Majesty the Queen Mother herself. In the midst of such reflections La Señora's attention is diverted by the sight of a Scotsman, handsomely kilted for the royal occasion. She is overcome.

'Ask him please if I may buy his skirt,' she directs me.

'No,' I reply, with uncustomary firmness. 'I will introduce you and you yourself may enquire about the availability of his kilt.'

So I do and she does.

'No,' says the handsome Scotsman with uncustomary uncertainty. 'Not this one, not tonight. May I introduce you to my wife?'

'What happened next?' I ask La Señora.

'He told me that I was a woman after his heart and I said well, I know what I am after. Then I felt it was time for a change in the conversation. So I twinkle the eye and I ask him "Do you sing?" "No, not so much," he replies. Then I ask if he likes Japanese food. Well, I do, but he says no, so I say no, I don't either. But all the time I was thinking that I wanted to buy his socks as well as his skirt. He was very young, like a pigeon. Anyway, you may buy for me some and I will love my Scottish socks and skirt that are coming.'

Kilts and pigeons aside, in near retrospect La Señora is so entirely seized by the depthless grandeur and majesty of the occasion that, almost forthwith, she passes long hours in her atelier decorating an ostrich egg with obscure, saintly medieval motifs and adorning the whole with gemstones, diamonds, pearls and rubies. The carpenter is then charged to construct a handsome box of appropriate dimensions in the topmost timber, imperceptibly dovetailed, and in turn the *obra maestra*, the Embellished Egg, is despatched post haste to Clarence House, London, England, no less, to be graciously received and graciously acknowledged.

There are other moments to savour. We are at a glittering engagement gathering – not that Peruvians ever need much of an excuse for a party. Nor do we need Hermogenic reminders of the philosophical and practical verity that engagements lead to weddings, thus provoking christenings. I am in the verdant garden by the poolside under the softly illuminated palms, innocuously sniffling the tropical night air and waiting for the Doctor to report back from his sortie to see if the pianist can play the Harry Lime theme, coupled with a surreptitious reconnaissance to locate the whereabouts of the chocolates. Waiters pass with gold-rimmed plates abundantly arranged with delicacies and yet more flutes of champagne. On the far side of the pool the band plays on under the *toldo*, the gracefully crêpe-draped awning erected for the dancers.

'Sit to me here and talk to me in my dinner,' I am bidden huskily by a hungry lady with hungry eyes. 'Make me company. I am imagining that you might be amongst the oddly qualified of this world. I think that perhaps you have had a very large life. To accommodate a large life you need a large heart. I can tell you that I gave my husband all my heart. I needed my heart to be very well welcome.'

So I sit. I have a feeling I might be on the menu. Lightly grilled with a touch of sauce, sunny side up. Now I realize that I have fleetingly seen my new companion previously, emerging from the Doctor's *consultorio* in the Clinic on sundry past occasions, although this is the first time we have spoken.

'Who is your name?' I am asked. The hungry lady leans her décolletage towards me to receive the answer.

I reveal my name, just the two four-letter words, unadorned and reassuring. In return I am presented with a life story. It's all in the name, you see. Uncomplicated. It inspires confidences, the sharing of the most profound secrets of the night.

'This evening you have to know all my life. I was marriaged to that green man over there, oof, many, many years ago. Now I am not. You may never trust a man in the first word. He was poor. I thought I will help him not to be poor. I spent my life waiting for my husband in the window. I learnt that he just wanted to come home to a palace done by who knows who. He had me as an object of art in his house. I was like a flower that you never put a drop of water to. He was my king, I never had such a high person in my life. "Thank you for letting me love you," I told him, "thank you for being you." Sometimes with his profession he travelled. Before he left I would say this to him. "Give me your hand. I need to touch your fingers. Let me touch your fingers one by one so that I might remember you, your heart and your soul, whilst you are gone. If I touch your face and your soul, it fills my heart so much."' Unknowingly, the hungry lady touches my hand in the sadness of her memories and we share the silence that ensues.

'Sometimes my husband might remember to ask of me on his return, "And how was your time whilst I was away?" "Oh, quite fine, thank you," I would say. "But of course, without you, not exceptional." Often in the days after he came home from one of his travels I would go with beating heart to the study where he worked at his papers. "Yes?" he would enquire, looking up from his desk and greeting me as one would a stranger. "Oh," I would reply, the words tripping on the lump in my throat, "I just came to see that you are still here,

147

I am so happy that you are home again, the pleasure of having your hand in mine." And he would smile a distant smile and return to his work. The smile was not for me. Maybe humiliation is the right word, maybe it is not, but I know that it was pain beyond pain.'

Once again we share the silence of the moment. Then from the depths of her bruised being she sighs and continues.

'And you, my new friend of this evening, as a man you may have many qualities but the scale and compass of such love is far beyond your comprehension. For you will know that whilst a man merely thinks, a woman feels. If my husband had kept me he would be double-priced. For many years I was opening the doors and windows of his life but he forgot me. He had many lovers. "It must be beautiful to be disputed by so many people," I told him. "We must be about five or six in your group. Maybe more. For me it is too many, I do not wish to share. I do not want even to share you with the wind that ruffles your hair." That man he taught me many things. At our end I said to him, "Please, the last teach: teach me how to leave you for ever and do it now please. Teach me well and I shall try my first steps alone to see if I fall. Then one day if you chance to see me passing, you can ask me, are you going well?" Now he is devalued and I wish that I had never met him. He was my evil. He destroyed my life. He should be sorry for what he did but that is not his way. May God grant that he will always sleep alone.' The curse of General Miller is carelessly cast in the direction of the green man before my confessor continues. 'You may think that love is a creative force. For me it was the opposite, it was a destructive force. Love is always joined with tears and sorrow. When you love you are infinitely richer but also you suffer. Nothing in this life on earth ever seems to be complete. But we can try and maybe still there is someone in this world that can be company for me. In twenty years I went to bed with my husband five times and I have six children.' Once again the hungry lady leans in my direction as the unbidden tears run silently down her cheeks. 'I was a forbidden person but now you will know that I too had a lover, although God sent him to my hands too late, even though in love there is no age. Love is the same in any age. Yes, after so many years I catch my feather and I said, "Now is not my moment, please wait for me." It was a grave mistake. I lost my feather. Now I am a changed person. I don't like to repeat, I like to change my dishes. Can you invite me a little wine, please? We will need the cork thing to pull up.'

'Yes, yes and yes,' I confirm.

'I am Catholic, but of course, I am not too Catholic. Do you believe in God? In your eyes I see an inner calm, internal peace and a life beyond.'

'Yes, I think so. Just in case. Everybody needs a religion, although not to the point of melancholia.'

'It is good to believe. We have a need to believe. There is a craving. I love people and I want to make people happy and I am living for that. I believe in God the only one, the one that gives the life and helps me to continue in this world. So I went to the priest for advice about my lover because I was not the divorcing kind. "Do you have a husband?" asked the priest. "Yes," I said. "And do you have children?" "Yes, many, great and small." "Do you love this other man?" "Yes, with all my heart, with all my soul." "Oh, we are so sorry for that. Do you want to see the Bishop? He is very in contact with these matters." "Oh, that would be too much," I said, "I just need to recovery back my soul." "In that case we would just recommend the application of recuperative time. Wait and see if things get better." So I said "thank you" and that was that and I left, carrying the pieces of my broken heart.'

I pull the cork and pour wine. We sip.

'I do not want to give you my age but maybe I am about fifty. In my other soul I am younger than what my age is. I am a poet, a poetess actually. Thankfully I have discovered that my life has another window. God, he took me something away but he gave me something back. God, be sure, will remember, even if sometimes he is late.'

I am not sure if I am following the conversation correctly. The hour is late as well as God. I look thoughtfully at the man in the green suit. Drink in hand, he appears normal, apart from the suit, of course. But behind closed doors? Once out of the green suit? Well, who can tell? One never knows. Maybe it was enough to drive a person to poetry.

'Never write with a computer,' comes the sudden warning from the hungry poetess. 'The personality is in the passage of the pen across the parchment, the softness of the strokes, the twists and turns of the letters, the boldness of the curls. The defiance of the flourishes. The caresses of the quill. The pulsing of the plume.'

'¡Caramba! Gosh! Have you published?'

'Please, no interruptions. The mind is in contact with the thoughts becoming words, passing to the paper. With the machine, it cuts the thinking. You lose the things. How do you feel?'

I feel as though I have lost my concentration for a moment. That's why people smoke pipes. Puff, puff, puff, tap, tap, push, suck, another puff. Playing for time. What was she talking about? Ah, the curl of the words. I nod solemnly; yes, I feel the same way.

'Now I want to speak goodbye to you.'

'Oh! Bye bye.' The conversational red card. Clearly I have failed to light a fire here. The price of inattention. I must try harder. But wait, the tragic poetess has one more thing to say to me.

'How is it that you came to end up here in Lima?' she enquires, her moist eyes replete with gentle perception. 'In this moment the hour is late but I do not wish to leave the night without an answer. Here in this country we have room and love for you. But why are you sitting in this country? That is what I am asking myself.'

My word! It's that statement again, masquerading as a question. And the answer? Well, how should I know? It's all a matter of wind and tide.

'When I am next in the Clinic,' says the hungry poetess, 'we may talk again.'

Once again the décolletage inclines. Now I sense the wind is freshening.

'Don't worry,' La Señora reassures me. 'That person she talks but she doesn't say anything. She just talks. She is a woman. She doesn't know what she is saying. She is nice but she is not capable. She is good for answering the telephone, nothing more. She knows her limits. Once upon a time she was always the most intelligent of the night. Now she is second hand, shrunk worse than an *huaca*, an adobe pyramid, a mouldy pile of dust. It is very known that she should go to the psychiatrist, very known. It is like the muffler is broken.'

Just then, Dr Hermogenes emerges cautiously from the shadow of the palm fronds.

'No luck with the Harry Lime theme,' he reports, shaking his head, reconnaissance mission completed. 'The curious thing was, when the pianist stopped to see if he had the music, the piano continued playing. In any case, the band say they haven't got a zither. But I've located the coffee creams. Follow me.'

At about this time, La Señora is also given to lapses in concentration.

'Remembering is not my best thing,' she is fond of telling us. 'I am short-minded.'

But there is more to it than that. La Señora is preoccupied with the World Ice Sculpture Championships in Sweden.

'I am extremely happily nervous about this trip,' she declares. 'With so much snow, I will have to wear a pair of those long shoes.'

'Long shoes?'

'Yes, those long shoes.'

'Ah, skis!'

'Call them what you like.'

It is my turn to reassure. 'Anyway, don't worry. While you are gone everything will be fine in the Clinic. Every corner kept immaculate, with lots of fresh flowers.'

'What?'

'I mean that we, Dr Hermogenes and I and Señorita Hilda and Ernestina and Nurse Dulce, we will all work our very hardest to keep the patients and the Bank happy. And that includes Dr Cleeber and Dr Ching. And Dr Vonday, of course.'

'Who? What about Dr Desastre?'

'Even him.'

Working in the medium of ice is slightly outside the everyday scope of most Peruvian artists, so the same informal committee that gave birth to The Tortured Nude is reconvened to conceive creative suggestions for a prize-winning Peruvian theme for the sculpturing competition. The final consensus is for an epic piece entitled 'Pisco Sour with Ice (without Pisco Sour)'. The committee is well pleased with this spectacularly droll inspiration, combining as it does a subtle blend of national pride, history and, well, many other virtues; La Señora is less impressed. She makes an independent declaration of intent concerning her theme. The style will be abstract. No further details are revealed, but that should cover all eventualities, including any inadvertent lurch of the slippery chisel on the yet-to-be-chipped exhibit. Very shrewd, but what will the judges opine? No doubt everything will be fine on the day and whatever the outcome it seems probable that at the next Christmas waifs and strays party, the Russian legacy will be joined by a Swedish contingent.

To share the general excitement and sense of adventure, the work of the committee is extended to advising on what to pack for the great ice odyssey. The Doctor declines his nomination for the packing advisory panel. He is still scarred by the memory of those rusty storks he carried round Europe on his honeymoon nearly thirty years ago. But he looks in from time to time to review progress.

'Let's see how is doing the Madam,' he says, casting his eyes round the room.

Chinese takeaways are sent for, a packing list is prepared, and then, on the eve of departure, the list is lost. The committee opens another bottle to debate this turn of events, whilst to set the scene and further lighten the mood, La Señora dons a Viking helmet, complete with horns, handily available from the family fancy-dress box. Packing reverts to the time-honoured system of wandering round the dishevelled dressing room wondering what to take.

'I do not wish you to see that I am a person with disorder in my life,' observes La Señora, as the Ice Cube Committee members review the contents of their glasses and studiously examine their boots.

La Señora's Great Circle route from Lima to Sweden, and coincidentally round and round the dressing room, contains several surprises. In goes the long red dress for dinner with friends in Madrid, in goes the long black dress for dinner with the Ambassador in Paris, in goes the long silver dress for dinner with the family in Estocolmo, all with matching shoes and accessories. Plus one of the mink coats. The only drawer in the wardrobe which is ignored is the large one, dedicated exclusively to La Señora's unique collection of rare and exotic bikinis, blessedly out-of-season for this excursion.

'Estocolmo, in three days you know the city like your house,' says La Señora, freely selecting another dress, just in case. 'On my travel I shall wear mainly black to shrink my weight.'

'Is this a fashion show or an Ice Sculpture Competition,' enquires one rash member of the committee.

The ensuing silence is indeed icy.

'Be careful, no? I am very busy in this moment. Very rushed,' warns La Señora. 'When we are in Paris we will go to the window of Chanel to see the latest fashions. We look very carefully with our eyes and when we return we make a copy.' Then she melts slightly. 'This is my hammer for working the ice,' she explains, brandishing, appropriately enough, a hammer. 'These are my goggles, against the flying pieces. Really for swimming, intelligent, yes? I just need to make a hole in the nose for the breathing. This is my *chuyo*, my traditional Peruvian hat from the high Andes. *Desafortunadamente*, I cannot see when I am wearing the goggles and the *chuyo*.'

With one accord our minds flick back to the abstract theme.

'Don't laugh at me, please. Here is my Peruvian poncho. And here are my Peruvian presents, little llamas and mountain pipes for the people.'

There, everything done, everything packed and prepared. Just three suitcases for the outbound trip. Always disregard the adage about only taking half of what you think you need. But in La Señora's case, definitely take twice as much money. At the very last moment a messenger arrives, or possibly a *correo electronico*, with details of the accommodation arrangements in Sweden, at the inventively and picturesquely named Arctic Hotel. The title is too evocative, too chilling for the warm-blooded embryonic ice sculptress.

'I think the weather will be very cold and I will shake a lot in the shower. I will definitely need the second mink coat,' she decides. 'Now, in this moment I have to take everything out and make it back.'

So we do. We repack. We are two hours late arriving at the airport. *La hora Señora*. Luck is on our side, the flight is also two hours late. La Señora has been known to miss flights. More than once: most recent in the memory is the occasion when she was supposedly nipping down to Santiago to breathe happiness over a Chilean wedding. But today all is well and she is in upbeat form.

'A dark wind and a dark day,' she says dramatically to the *watchiman* at the airport barrier, leaning out of the car window. 'There will be a *temblor*.' And we drive on, leaving the prophecy hanging ominously in the exhaust fumes.

'Why did you tell him that about an earthquake?' I ask. 'You just made that up.'

'Yes, just to frighten him. But if we have one he will be so proud of knowing me.'

The departure of La Señora has attracted a substantial group of well-wishers. There is much embracing and excited talk amongst the members of the party, none of it related to the departing heroine. It is the way of farewell gatherings in Peru, the send-off group are usually so immersed in their private conversations that everybody forgets why they came and the traveller often leaves unnoticed, the bugles unsounded. Although not in La Señora's case, of course.

'I am wearing this special scent,' she informs us poignantly, hushing the chatter. 'It is called "Remember Me". Now you have to know who I am when I return.'

It is time to go, time to board the flight, Europe-bound. Back to the Old World, farewell to El Nuevo Mundo. Time to say goodbye, good luck. We love you. Come back safely, come back soon.

'This trip will be fun and easy,' declares La Señora bravely. Then, being a true artist, she quotes Degas for us. '"Everyone has what it takes to fail. To succeed is a far harder thing."' With that, and a swirl of the mink, she is gone. Off to the frozen north.

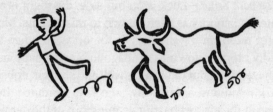

14

El Festival de Taurino y La Pamplonada

Thus, without so much as a backward glance, La Señora takes flight and temporarily abandons us to our toil in the Clinic whilst merrily she chips abstract ice cubes in the opposite hemisphere on what seems to us to be the far side of the globe. For the stay-at-homes in Lima, Peru, it is a question of following the cosmic dictates of the passage of the sun as best we can in our deprived circumstances and of filling our days with whatever crumbs of comfort and joy chance to pass our way. In the Clinic our remit is clear: up the income, down with expenditure. More promotion, more patients, fewer shopping trips. *Sin commentario*, as they say in these parts. Count the pennies, or rather the nuevos soles, and try to keep up with the payments on the loan. That aside, it just so happens that fortune is with us, for happily this is the *época* of *El Festival de Taurino* in the old bullring of the abandoned hacienda at Cañete.

The Doctor is in his element. He makes the necessary arrangements. The bravest matadors and the strongest *toros* are engaged for the gala occasion. The supporting cast of *los subalternos*, twiddling their off-season thumbs in the city, arrive from Plaza de Acho. They all come, inseparable, even the unloved picador, with welcoming fanfares and brass accompaniment provided by the enthusiastic musicians of Cañete. Meanwhile, back in Miraflores, Dr Vonday straightens with pride, disturbs the dust from his ever-ready consulting couch, dons a fresh white coat and joins Manolo the unvigilant *vigilante* on the sunny front doorstep of the Clinic, awaiting trade like barber and son on a slack day for shaving and trimming.

Under the Doctor's aegis, the complex and historic tapestry that is *los toreos*, the bullfights, is woven into the renovated bull-ring of a bygone era and the stage is set for a true gem of an event. And so it is. The little-known, private Cañete occasion combines all the traditional ingredients of the tournament: ceremony, colour, grace, agility, courage and skill, and a classic miniature edition of the contentiously evocative spectacle of bullfighting is enacted in the environs of the deserted hacienda.

The Cañete version of *La Pamplonada* a few days later, the bull run based on and borrowed from the famous fiestas of San Fermín, is equally traditional but more informal. Oh yes, I am advised, we do this every year and everyone takes part. Of course. Just wear any old clothes and some running shoes. Ah yes, running shoes. Medical Student One helpfully explains the history of the event.

'The original run in Pamplona dates from the fourteenth century and stemmed from the need to take the fighting bulls from the Santo Domingo corrals to the actual Bull Ring. And then, no doubt, the practice became a test of manhood for the youth of the town.'

'No doubt,' I reply, doubtfully, inwardly debating the relevance of this test to me.

Unfinished with his erudition, Medical Student One moves from practice to theory.

'The human can run as fast as the bull,' he tells me.

I never knew that before. Is my mentor perfectly sure of this? All humans? Me?

'So, you just jog along with the bulls, preferably just in front if you like.'

I think I do like.

'And it looks better if you have a rolled newspaper and just tickle the nose of the bull as you pass along.'

Pass along? Or pass away? Does it have to be *El Comercio* of the day in question, or just any old newspaper?

'Don't you worry about the details, we'll all be there, same as every year.' And Medical Student Two nods with unconvincing vigour to confirm the veracity of Medical Student One's pronouncements.

I arrive at the appointed place at the appointed hour. Old clothes, running shoes. I have decided against the newspaper; perhaps a little too showy for my first outing. There is no sign of the Medical Students or the Doctor yet, but there is a fair gathering for the event. The majority, I now note, are not in running shoes and are standing behind a barrier erected at one side of the dusty track. On the other side is a crumbling dusty wall. I judge that the run itself must be about 500 metres, including a sharp right-angle bend, which appears to be the favoured viewing site for most of the spectators. The advertised hour comes and goes and as I stand waiting in the hot sun along with a handful of other intrepid sportsmen, all about one third my age, I am overcome with an increasing sense of déjà vu. I expect the vultures will be along in a moment.

At *la hora peruana*, precisely, a large truck appears at the end of the track, full of bellowing bulls. Full-sized, fed-up, bellowing bulls. By this time the spectator stands are packed and the number of what may be termed contenders has grown to some fifty or sixty. Apart from the Medical Students, and the Doctor, yes, it does seem that everyone is here, mostly situated on the safe side of the barriers. My sense of déjà vu is replaced by a familiar feeling of wishing that I could be somewhere else. Anywhere.

A shout goes up and down the track I see that the bulls are on the move. This is it, *La Pamplonada* is under way. Ah good, now I spot my senior mentor, Dr Hermogenes. But what's this? He is behind the herd, and no, I don't believe what I am seeing. But yes, the wicked Doctor is actually engaged in firing rockets. Can you can credit that? Not distress rockets. I could use one of those. The Doctor is firing loud banging go-faster rockets to hasten the stampeding bulls on their way. Towards us, that is. Mentor or tormentor?

Under close questioning later in the day the Doctor insists that the rockets are standard San Fermín signals to inform interested parties (like me, I suppose) that, first, the gates are open. Secondly, the bulls have left and their presence is imminent (I think I guessed that). Thirdly, 'the bulls have entered the taurine enclosure' (no one told me about that, I didn't know we had one). Fourth and final rocket: 'the beasts have gone into the bullpens and the Bull Run is over' (for the benefit of any surviving runners, I imagine). I squint hard and sceptically at the Doctor.

But for the moment, panic has gripped my fellow contestants. Me too. We are off on our own stampede, no rockets needed. I have that familiar feeling of my feet being beyond my control. Morro Solar, *La Capea*, Carnival, here we go again. In years to come when people ask me what I thought of Peru, I shall tell them.

'Good running country,' I shall say. Never mind the Incas. Or Machu Picchu.

More immediately, things are getting serious again. For I am trailing the youthful pack of stampeding humanity. The snorting bellowing herd of rocket-assisted bulls, encouraged by the evil Doctor, is drawing ever closer. Medical Student One is incorrect with his information. Some human beings cannot run as fast as a bull. I am one of them. If ever I see Medical Student One again I shall inform him of his error. It seems that not even a tightly rolled copy of *El Comercio* can save me now, and I prepare, yet again, to meet my Maker. One thing that Medical Student One omitted to tell me is that between 1924 and 1997 a total of fourteen souls perished in the Pamplona run, with more than two hundred people injured by the bulls. The gift of total recall in one's final moments is a well-known phenomenon.

I pray for a miracle. It is my last resort. Just as swiftly, and indeed miraculously, a miracle comes my way. A leather-faced gentleman appears at my elbow. Moving easily, he gives me a smile and a nod. My new friend has twinkling eyes, deep set in his nut-brown countenance, about as useful as my twinkling toes at this moment of truth, as the bulls lower their horns and move in for the kill.

'Step this way,' says the miracle man coolly, as we swing together round the right-angle bend in the concourse, the packed crowd blurred but intent.

So saying, he pulls me into a hidden niche in the crumbling wall running beside the track.

'There,' he says comfortingly, as the bulls thunder past harmlessly, deprived of their quarry. We step out nonchalantly into the dust cloud hanging over the now deserted track to view the departing stampede of youth and bulls.

'They will be back soon,' advises the leather-faced man, with another twinkle. 'Follow me.'

True, back come the bulls, preceded by the dusty puffing youths. We take our time, fearlessly sauntering round the corner, dicing with death. The crowd shrieks for our safety but we are masters of the situation. A light tug on my arm, a neat shimmy of the hips and there we are, secure in a second niche. We watch the grumpy bulls lollop past, thwarted again, and we take centre stage to see them into the distance.

'See you next year,' twinkles my saviour, and he is gone before I can pump his arm and slap his back. The power of prayer.

I stroll down to the beach house, just in time to see Medical Student Two disappearing towards the ocean, happy surfboard under his arm. Medical Student One emerges blinkingly into the unfamiliar sunlight, carrying a rolled copy of *El Comercio*.

'Where have you been?' he asks, politely uninterested.

'To hell and back,' I answer lightly.

'Oh.' And unimpressed with the brightness of the day he returns to his bed. With his rolled newspaper, just in case.

Then, appropriately, with the end of Carnival, *La Capea*, *La Pamplonada* and the accompanying festivities, with the departure of La Señora to the North Pole, or near by, the summer sun deserts the golden sands and the weather fades. The colourful Cañete beach umbrellas and cheerful towels are furled and folded for another year and, subdued and silent, each with his own thoughts and sun-filled memories, we drive back to autumnal Lima, soon to become wintry Lima the Grey, as though the seaside interlude was but a fast-fading fantasy. Our pervading preoccupations for the future of the Clinic are inescapable.

Journeying along the overcrowded highway, the life-threatening Pan Americana Sur, with its plethora of toll stops and rows of stalls selling all the things for the beach that nobody will want for another year, we see that the silent beauty of the arid moonscape mountains has indeed been mindlessly desecrated with huge graffiti in readiness for the forthcoming presidential elections. The repetitive political slogans have all been executed with commendable military precision; no need to call in calligraphy experts with a magnifying glass to read the clue. Like it or not, our passive political involvement is unavoidable: the economic slump under the current regime is affecting both sides of the Clinic's survival equation. Patient numbers are being depressed; interest rates are astronomical. Our summer's end return to Lima is truly a return to reality.

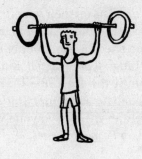

15

Merengues Peruanos

The workaday calm of the Clinic, customarily crisply effi- cient and smoothly subdued, is disturbed by Señorita Hilda, uncharacteristically agitated. Eagerly anticipated, word is in from the World Ice Sculpture Championships, via outer space and the internet. The Incas used stalwart *chasquis* running timelessly with a cleft stick. More reliable. Nevertheless, impa- tiently we gather round Señorita Hilda's desk to scan the screen for cosmic confirmation that La Señora has been crowned Ice Sculpting Champion of Planet Earth and Queen of the Frozen North. We read the text excitedly but can't believe our eyes.

'Don't forget to feed Carlotta.' That's the message. Feed the tortoise! Is that all? Oh, all right.

Everybody drifts back to whatever they were doing and to wherever they were doing it. Nobody feeds Carlotta. Then more news filters through, although it is not exactly as we had hoped. No Gold Medal for La Señora, at least, not with the hammer and chisel. Possibly with the iced cocktails. But out of the countries taking part, we learn that the Peruvian representatives have

163

been nominated as finalists on their very first occasion of competing. *¡Caray!* No one is quite clear what that implies, least of all Nurse Dulce who sheds a tear, but definitely it must have been a close-run thing. *¡Qué triunfo!* But best to withhold further comment until the Ice Cube Committee can be reformed to hear and debate our competitor's first-hand report. Or until the unlikely event that anyone chances to see the promised coverage on *People and Arts*.

In the wider world of entertainment, the rigged Peruvian presidential elections draw ever closer, marked not by apathy, not by indifference, but by a strong sense of the ineluctable. Human rights groups and other worthy bodies visit the country and from the forecourts of the best hotels declare as one that '*No existen condiciones para elecciones libres y transparentes*'. Then they pack and leave, and after the huffing and the puffing, life continues unchanged.

'What happens now?' I ask over lunch with Dr Hermogenes, focusing on the unanimous observation that 'conditions for free and transparent elections are non-existent'.

'Nothing. Why?'

'Oh, I just wondered.'

'Wondered what?'

'Well, that perhaps . . . '

'In this country we do not ask questions to which we do not know the answers.'

The dark side of Peru. Before 1980, twelve years of military dictatorship destroyed the economic infrastructure of the country, in particular the vital strand of agriculture. For the next ten years the return to democracy under two increasingly ineffectual presidencies was accompanied by the appearance of terrorist groups, an explosion in drug trafficking and soaring inflation, matched only by the growth of governmental corruption. The decade of the 1990s brought an unchanged President, a stagnant economy, terrorism on the wane and corruption on the gain. As the years passed, the centralized grip of the President on government and power became ever tighter.

In a masterstroke of electioneering the incumbent President, and presidential candidate, 'solves the problem' of *los invasores* by promising a plot of land to all Peruvian non-landowners. Free. Just line up and sign. Predictably, the happy voters do exactly that, at the rate of 20,000 a day. The other presidential candidates are left trailing in the slipstream, united only by heavy breathing and hot air.

There are seven or eight of the 'also-rans', nine including invisible Ezequiel, the white-bearded octogenarian. His electoral plank is an afforestation programme for *la costa*, so on the basis of voting for the man promising least, Ezequiel should be in with a shout. Except that as he shuns publicity on religious grounds, his campaign is impeded and in the opinion polls he maintains a depressingly consistent half per cent of the popular vote. In any case, the revelation in *El Comercio* that some one million false signatures have been added to the electoral roll on behalf of the President (and presidential candidate), together with several thousand ineligible military names, appears to put the whole issue safely beyond doubt. No one seems surprised at the disclosure, just slightly cross with *El Comercio*, that admirable and brave newspaper, for publishing such unsettlingly unnecessary news.

Meanwhile, in the micro-world of our equally admirable pile-carpeted Clinic, the albatross of our building loan hangs as a dead weight on the mildly eccentric shoulders of the absentee management. In response to our entreaties the Bank devises a new finance plan that will, on analysis, cost even more than our existing terms, and our banker, owner of the famously Tortured Nude, affects to be startled when we spot the trick and decline to sign. Conversely, down in Cañete we gladly affirm an agreement with the *Alcade*, the local Mayor, to construct a charitable primary healthcare centre for the needy people of that area, largely lying beyond the short reach of state provision. But, we have to explain, be patient please until we find a way to stop the Bank from taking all our income, for only then can we implement the noble dreams of La Señora, which with time-honoured idealism will propel the reluctant rich to assist the struggling poor. Find a way we must, for the sands of time are running out along with the money.

Our patient numbers appear to have reached a plateau, not that any scientific market analysis data are to hand; quite simply, the capricious daily peaks and troughs are averaging out to much the same total at the end of every month. Dr Desastre continues to minister to a breathless puff of rotund visitors and Dr Cleeber is forever active in the theatre, trimming and sculpting. But without the lift to give easy access to the upper floors, we are still without in-patients and Dr Hermogenes is obliged to conduct his deliveries in other clinics and hospitals.

High on the agenda for La Señora's return must be the urgent need to consider once again the disposal of a few assets to reduce our borrowing. Maybe a car or two could be sacrificed or even perhaps the unvisited family smallholding at Huachipa, where the forgotten and unlamented Programa de Investigación de Hortalizas Exóticas and the Centro de Investigación y Producción de Endivias de Bruselas 'Witloof' have both long ceased to flourish. Possibly, thinking the unthinkable in accordance with the best management manuals, even the desert farm should go under the hammer.

Meanwhile, it is not the South American way to be despondent.

'The country does not exist with such a diversity of food as Peru,' says the Doctor. 'It is our duty to partake. The coastal cuisine has its emphasis on fish and other seafood, accompanied by rice, lime and onion, yucca and chicken and pork. The cuisine of *la sierra*, the Andean cuisine, uses lamb and porks with potatoes, sweet corn and other grains, with trout from the mountain streams. Whilst the cuisine of the rainforest includes freshwater fish such as the huge *paiche* of the Amazon and the smaller dorado; alligator and turtle are served with heart of palm and rice, and then come all the tropical fruits of the region.'

That's the beauty of subjective judgements. The Doctor and Mr Nobody, gourmet and gourmand, elevated to being the world's leading authorities. The Incas, the Spanish with their Arab cooks and Negro slaves, the French, the Italians and the Orientals: all have contributed to the culinary delights to be sampled in Peru. Less so the British. They made more impact in the struggle for Independence than in the battle for honours in the kitchen.

We fall easily into our gastronomic routine, readily adjustable to accommodate the erratic vagaries and demands of the Doctor's morning appointments. There are days when Nurse Dulce, brimming with suppressed pride, is able to present a full page of activity; other days, for no discernible reason, the telephone scarcely rings and the eager diary remains discarded and disappointed on the desk. Come what may, on completion of his schedule of unpredictable patients, often late, rarely early, and his equine obligations, the Doctor rings my office on the top floor of the Clinic.

'Are you hungry enough?' he enquires rhetorically, and off we go. He knows every restaurant of repute in Lima and, in the lengthening absence of La Señora, wending homewards via the capitals of Europe, what can we do but put his knowledge to the test? 'Yes,' he says happily when his memory has served him well. 'I remember this place. See how they place a good-looking chicken on the door to call the attention of the people to try their hen soup. It is the best. Here we may also find an ancestral appetizer from the Incas.'

So we eat our *caldos*, *chupes* and cream soups, we sample the celebrated *cebiches* based on raw fish marinaded in lemon juice, we eat potatoes and rice tasting better by far than all others, ever, anywhere. Then, by way of change we try *camote*, *yuca*, *oca* and *maca*, the edible root crops of the country. To the latter, the Peruvian ginseng, are attributed remarkable fortifying powers.

'This aphrodisiac comes from the high mountains,' Dr Hermogenes explains, helpfully, 'although attempts to culti- vate it in the Himalayas have not met with success.' Whilst on the subject of medicinal plants, the Doctor also extols the virtues of *la uña de gato*, prepared from the bark of a jungle creeper of the same name, booster for the immune system and possessing unequalled anti-inflammatory powers for the treat- ment of arthritis and rheumatism and now the subject of much medical interest.

For working lunches, on those days when Nurse Dulce, prompted by the arbitrary call of the erratic diary, is gently per- suasive in curtailing our lunch hour or when Ernestina's noughts and grease spots are demanding audit, the Doctor is an adherent of *mondongo*, a dish of tripe, entrails, beef and corn, or he advocates *causa*, based on the yellow potato, mashed with tuna, crab or chicken. From the abundance of ocean seafood we eat oysters and other shellfish, shrimps and lob- sters, whilst of all the available varieties of fish, *corvina* and *len- guado* are our favourites, together with those mountain river trout. With his well-honed surgical skills, the Doctor is an excellent dissecter.

'Here is the most tasteful part,' he is fond of explaining. 'This is a very fresh fish. He is also accompanied by fresh vegetables. And here is another food. I hope you will like the knee of the pork that I am inviting you.'

At weekends we enjoy fine light Ocucaje and Tacama, best of the Peruvian wines, deriving from Ica, the country's wine capital 300 kilometres south of Lima. Or there are Cristal, Cusqueña and Arequipeña beers to be sampled and we are grateful for the blessed inheritance of the siesta. On other occasions we eat more frugally from roadside stalls, *arroz zambito*, *mazamorra morada*, *champus*: black rice pudding made with *chancaca* unprocessed sugar; dark red maize boiled with the flour of the sweet potato with ginda berries and dried peaches; *champus* consisting of hot stewed fruit, mainly *guanabana* and pineapple, corn soup and other magical ingredients.

From afar we are nudged by the nutritional hand of La Señora and we heed her advice.

'Whilst I am gone to the ice be sure that you are well fed. I want to feed you well but at this time I must depend on you. You need to decide if you will eat in function of your appetite or only in function of your brain. Either way, on my return I do not wish to find you in famine condition. In restaurants it is best to order a lot. We never know when it is our last dinner. Remember how good and fresh is a Peruvian salad and also that soups are very dietful. These will make your stomachs very happy. You never met a person that loves soups as I do. As soon as we have patients staying in the Clinic I shall personally be arranging their menus, with Dr Desastre of course, to expedite their immediate recovery. A long time ago I heard the story of the stone soup and I still believe in that soup. For preparing hen soup of course you will need a piece of hen. This is a soup that is very tasteful. You must boil the water as hot as you can, that is the soup secret. Our Peruvian seafood is also very dietful but he who talks and eats a fish can die. For me, I find the *corvina* can be a very emotional fish, *sí*? When I eat one I think everyone is looking to me and waiting to see the results.'

When we have over-indulged, La Señora is again at our elbow.

'First you could eat an elephant, then you are very happy full and now is the moment to walk your rice and your fullness, especially if your onions are in a revolution and you are struggling with your stomach. And never neglect the soufflé which takes just ten minutes to be done. It is very French.'

Our sense of deprivation at being without the presiding presence of La Señora is serendipitously softened by the proximity of Dasso, urban village within a city, the Notting Hill of Lima. A few blocks from the Clinic, a day can be lost in Village Dasso, even a lifetime, and there need be no cause to travel further. It has everything. Shops of all descriptions, banks, laundries, restaurants, pavement cafés, coffee stalls, ice cream parlours, Turkish baths and gymnasia for bodily well-being, nearby churches for spiritual health, a casino to expedite financial ruin and finally a funeral parlour for use when the time is nigh, bereft of money, incapacitated and incapable. Swept away on the uncertain currents of faith, hope and charity. Pending that day, Dasso also has an unimaginable number of *peluquerías* to give an unimagined variety of hair styles. It is here that Dr Hermogenes takes his cautious monthly cut, and where with equal regularity the crimper conspiratorially confides his confident conviction that, rain or shine, hairdressers and gynaecologists alike share a common bond in that they will never lack the necessary, considering the vital service that each provides to humanity.

Concrete is the substance of Dasso, the buildings and banks, the shops and apartment blocks; from the denizens of Dasso springs the soul of that microcosmic subculture. Every day sees the same pavement politicians sitting outside the same coffee shops; the unvarying elderly and infirm clutching tartan rugs over their knees as they are perambulated in the sunshine by their faithful, white-starched dusky nurses; the familiar stall holders and *ambulantes*, the street vendors; the cloned ultra-elegant ladies of a certain age from a lost epoch taking coffee, taking tea, talking, talking; the passing tourists with their enormous bulging backpacks and incongruous Darkest Africa khaki safari shorts, like big-game hunters who mistakenly took the wrong flight. Darkest Wildest Africa, Deepest Darkest Peru: easily done.

'Why are there so many people here selling calculators?' ask the bemused tourists in their confused safari shorts. And the pavement politicians sitting outside the cafés have to explain that, no, it's not quite like that, these people in the red surcoats are after your money, they are *cambistas*, calculator-waving money-changers, ever active in Dasso, anxious for trade, seven days a week. So much so that whenever you leave the bank they are insistently at your side.

'*¿Cambio? ¿Cambio?*' Change? Change?

There are just two currencies on offer, dollars and nuevos soles. Why is it that *los cambistas* imagine that you are so light in the head that every time you make a bank transaction you inadvertently do so in the wrong currency with the result that on leaving the premises you immediately need to change the entire contents of your wallet?

It is the same convoluted logic that leads the extra-energetic *lustrabotas*, the middle-aged boot-boys in their wooden cubicles, to offer an immaculate shine for your suede shoes, and similarly leads the perverse Tico *taxistas* to offer you a lift when you are patently jogging in a tracksuit or merely trying to cross the road. 'Beep, beep', they go, 'beep, beep', worse than the yellow peril of the D'Onofrio ice cream hordes.

No one in their right mind travels in a Tico taxi anyway: people leaving them try to look invisible, as though they have just come out of the bathroom. 'I am not here; I was not in

171

there.' Four aspects of Tico-travelling are unfailingly dependable. First, your life will be in acute danger; second, you will be overcharged; third, the driver will be unable to find your destination; fourth, reveal you are from London and wait to be rewarded: 'England?' Pause. 'Bobby Charlton!'

Combis too. No one admits to travelling in a combi, especially wearing a jacket and tie. The hailing trick is to look blankly in the opposite direction until the ultimate moment when an almost imperceptible flicker of the eye, or a lift of the big toe, is sufficient to pass the necessary message to the kamikaze *chofer*, he of the rocket-like reactions, so that without warning his mini-bus surges across the traffic from the outside lane, braking hard and oblivious to all but the prospect of one more nuevo sol in the kitty. Then leap through the door quickly in the hope that no one has spotted you, like entering the chemist's on illicit business, urged on by the cries of the conductor, '¡*Sube, sube!* up, up!' Clever Incas. No combis or Ticos in *el Imperio Incaico*, the Inca empire. They were banned by imperial decree, a little-known fact. Along with yellow ice cream bicycles.

Everyone is watchful in Village Dasso, looking to learn everybody else's business. If sprawling, sighing Lima is a sad and suffering city of onomatopoeic *suspiros*, then Dasso is assuredly a festering mini-world of *susurros y chismoso*, whispers and gossip. Cross the road with one señorita and 'Ah hah!' say *los lustrabotas*. Return ten minutes later with another and 'Uh huh!' say *los cambistas*, punching two and two into their ever-optimistic calculators and making five whilst the net curtains of the local laundrette twitch and proprietor Señor Aurelianos looks meaningfully at his wife.

'*Sí*,' confirms proprietress Señorona Aniseta, 'he's watering the broccoli again.'

Village life: find out what you can, make up what you can't. The more uncomplimentary the better.

'This is Peru,' comes a knowing murmur from the frozen north. 'They have ears like an elephant, listening all the time meanwhile you are not there. The purest thing is not to be in the mouth of anyone but yourself. And never trust in confidantes; here they will put your life to the wall.'

Bizarre. Disconcerting too. It is almost as if La Señora knew that the Hungry Poetess had made good her undertaking to visit the fourth floor.

Body 2000 is the Dasso fitness centre, directly competing with the funeral parlour, or possibly affiliated. Typical of the genre, on three extensive floors it offers everything for the body beautiful, tantalizingly unattainable for most, with or without the caring, carving assistance of Doctors Desastre and Cleeber combined. Machines, apparatus and equipment to attend to every conceivable muscle, instructors at every turn to assess, advise and discreetly adjust.

'Are you fitted?' enquire the ladies, clad in their curvaceous leotards, many of whom are half recognizable from fleeting encounters in the Clinic.

'Yes, I'm fitted,' comes the response.

Non-stop classes in Spinning, Tae Bo, Aerobics, Exercise Dancing and more. Take your pick from Power Step, Fitness Step, Super Step, Circuit Step, Interval Step, Step Up, Cardio Training and Step *Avanzada. Definitivamente*, step this way for the body beautiful. Or the funeral parlour. To monitor progress, or regression, the *gimnasio* scales are so sensitive they can detect if you have had a pedicure or a hot-dog, a haircut or a hamburger. Gymnasium Body 2000 has everything that is anathema to La Señora. Nevertheless, she is prey to spontaneous bursts of enthusiasm, or remorse.

'My appear is not to my liking,' she declares on her late-morning arrival at the Clinic. 'I am strange. I look like a pork steak. In fact my facial cheeks are expanding out of normal borders.' Then she reflects. 'I am not like this, I am just temporarily like this. I do not know how this has occurred, I'm not a kind of desperate person if I see a big cake or something. In fact, there are some days when I do not have too much hunger. However, I need to lower the size of some of my aspects. Definitely soon I will be weighting less. But not too much, it is good to smile with round cheeks. However, today I am in a sports mood because last night I ate noodles.'

La Señora the artist is given to theatrical exaggeration. When the mood is upon her she pays her subscription. The following week, or earlier, she claims a refund. As is often the case with radical remedies, La Señora suffers severe side-effects from *el gimnasio*.

'Immediately after exercise I fall to sleep,' she explains on her return. 'Or I feel nauseating. And I spend more time in the changing room rearranging my hair than I do in the gymnasium. Today I have a pain in the shoulder and my downstairs legs have contractions. This *gimnasio* business is interrupting my life.'

A little while later we dutifully enquire after her state of health. Fortunately she is no longer nauseating and happily the shoulder is cured, along with the downstairs legs.

'That's a relief,' we chorus. 'Who cured you?'

'My dentist.'

'Your dentist?'

'Yes. He gave me a recipe and someone else gave me the injection.'

'Oh, good.' Best not to enquire further.

'Also I have these tablets which cause drowsness.'

'Do you enjoy this?' La Señora demands of the Body 2000 customers at large on those rare occasions that she mounts an exercise bicycle. 'Why is everyone so serious? Is it permitted to talk here?' Nobody answers. 'Everybody they just look at me. Oh, they think, poor woman, she doesn't even want to come. It is true, I am going against my volition. To lose the pizza it is easier to take a pill. This athletic behaviour is not for me.'

La Señora's conversation with the cosmopolitan clientele is about as satisfactory as mine.

'Finished?' I enquire with circumspect politeness of a man-mountain disengaging himself from a machine that I am hoping to put through its paces.

'No,' he says, looking down but equally politely. 'German.'

At least I got a reply.

Occasionally La Señora uses the running machines. Not for running, obviously. Arming herself with four or five assorted newspapers and fashion magazines, she first sets the contrivance to summer-day strolling speed. It's not marked on the dial but she can find it blindfold. Then she lays out her reading material on the control panel in front of her and relaxes.

'All the preoccupations are in the walking,' she explains.

'You know you can have a shower in the gym after your workout,' advises Medical Student One helpfully.

'Why?' queries the strolling Señora. 'I don't need a shower after reading the news, thank you. What kind of magazines do you think these are?'

Of course, it's an entirely different matter if you happen to have a personal fitness trainer, such as Statuesque Wellington Fisher from somewhere-in-the-Caribbean. After undergoing S. W. Fisher's personalized attentions, you probably need two showers, providing you can make it back to the changing room in the first place.

'In the body building you have to be aggressful,' Wellington tells his panting personal protégés, 'you must aggress dee bar. Then you get dee pomp.' The pumpy-pomp or the pompi-pump? Through some undefinable process of association I am reminded that we haven't started our Clinic classes yet, relaxation, general fitness, prenatal, post-natal.

Whatever, SWF's personal clients do as they are told and aggress dee bar, but still Statuesque Wellington asks for more.

'Hold the bar straight,' he insists, 'otherwise we build you up like an old boot. All down on one side.'

Even Wellington himself has his lopsided, lighter aspects.

'You look pretty snuffed out to me, ol' boy,' he encouragingly tells anyone on the point of collapse, male or female. Then as a further boost to morale he follows up with an illustrative anecdote. 'Training for dee National Championships, dose five-hundred-kilogram weights pin me down, man. Dee gravity he pull down dee bar, it was coming too much for me. But I aggress dee bar and fight dee gravity. And dose weights they don't pin me down no more.' Wellington Fisher playfully pumps his pecs and lengthens his lats.

'Beat dee drums and start dee dancing, heh man?'

And once again my thoughts turn to our under-utilized auditorium-cum-gymnasium.

Open seven days a week, the Body 2000 gym is a sad place on Saturdays and Sundays, a refuge for the heartless, filled with the ghosts of the departed Bodies-Beautiful. The cult is a circular vice. The Bodies-Beautiful toil away at their exercises during the week so that they will look good on the beach at the weekend whilst they get a tan so that they will look good in the gym during the week whilst they get ready for looking good on the beach to take their tan. The ultimate in self-fulfilling, self-perpetuating addictions.

La Señora: the archetypal disruptive influence, draped in a T-shirt emblazoned 'Fight Fizzical Fitness' in ultra-large letters. Who else would arrange personal delivery of a large box of cream-and-jam-filled doughnuts as I am furiously pedalling my bicycle in the middle of the packed Spinning class?

The mystery carton is marked 'Urgent – Open Now!' So I do, with the result that the forbidden treasures are exposed to the public gaze and a hand-written card from La Señora falls to the floor. Shock horror! I smile feebly at my fellow participants, but my credibility as a serious exponent of the sect of the body beautiful is in tatters. I hide the card from view but it is too late. Everybody has read the message: 'These cakes are very good and taste very happy. I think you never had cakes as fine as these.' I clutch my box defiantly and slink away to a corner to eat the sugar-coated doughnuts in solitude. No use trying to share with my contemptuous classmates. Delicious. All mine. But no more '¡*Holas!*' for me in *el gimnasio*. Never again. I am finished, a figure of fun, teased by the other boys; the girls pull my hair and pinch me.

Sybaritically speaking, *los baños turcos* in Dasso are more in La Señora's line, the non-physical, horizontal approach to fitness. More opportunities for chatting. The Turkish baths have many disciples and the cash register pings melodiously as the fat, fit, not-so-fat and not-so-fit come and go, in company with the out of shape, out of order and the completely collapsed.

It's all a matter of dedication. Even La Señora has transitory moments of apparent success, unlikely though this may seem, and whether the credit is due to the baths or the gym (or neither) is anyone's guess.

'Now today I am indeed weighting less,' she informs us, outwardly triumphant, inwardly as doubtful as we are. 'I lost the weight in the scales as well as in the looks.'

Overall, we have to accept that the gym is not for La Señora.

'I think this is boring. Boring. How did the Incas manage?' she wants to know.

She has a point there.

'Well . . . '

But she is not listening. Never listen to answers. They confuse. And anyway, they get in the way of the next question.

Unannounced, an expensive-looking rowing machine appears in the Clinic during La Señora's absence abroad, indubitably furtively ordered after lights-out from the pages of a health magazine. 'It is for the patients,' comes the casual explanation from the northern hemisphere in response to Señorita Hilda's telephone calls, convincing nobody, least of all the Doctor and his pregnant patients, and the chrome and black-padded folly is left to gather dust in a corner of the auditorium.

Seemingly without warning and quite catching us off our tranquil balance, the comfortable status quo of the placid and contented daily round in the Clinic and in the environs of Village Dasso is rudely disturbed. La Señora is reportedly in the stratosphere, airborne and homeward bound; imminent is her return to Peru, bearing those unquantifiable artistic accolades from the competitive furnace of the World Ice Sculpture Championships. Farewell to the culinary delights of our leisurely survey of Peruvian cuisine; farewell also, assuredly, to the mid-morning visits of the Hungry Poetess to bask in the creative calm of my fourth-floor office, bearing the fruits of her latest poetic inspirations. The predatory signature of her stressful tread on the stairs has become readily recognizable, taut and short, unlike the plump and accommodating footfalls of some of my other regulars.

'Read this,' says the Poetess, without preamble. 'I have written a piece for you. Actually, it is just the title at this point. "Lend me the Sky of your Eyes". In fact, perhaps it is a quotation; maybe you have heard of it? Possibly it is known. The rest will follow inspirationally, I may write a trilogy. I have a desire to embrace the symphonic harmonic combination of "Herculean" and "cerulean". How do you feel for that? Of course, the authorial problem, and this you may realize, is that we only have a finite number of words at our disposal and therefore sooner or later duplication is inevitable. There is a mathematical limitation to the number of permutations available to me as a poet. I have to hurry with my work because probably in Mongolia at this very moment someone is writing identically. For example, Shakespeare and Dickens were very fortunate to have been born so early. It was easy for them. Soon everything that is possible will have been written, the same will happen with music. It has already happened in the game of chess and possibly in cards as well. I do not watch football, but probably that too has almost exhausted itself, all the possible moves have been played and soon the spectators will watch a game and then realize that they have already seen it. Anyway, I must continue as best I can. Here is another poem that I am working on:

> "Sharing an evening and finding a friend
> Sharing friendship and finding love
> Sharing the world with our lives entwined
> Sharing the completeness of encircled love
> Enshrined in a fountain-filled courtyard
> Splashed with happiness under the wondering stars."

Do you think it is original?' she asks anxiously.

'You could call it "Sharing". I was wondering what time your appointment is with Dr Hermogenes?'

'And on this piece of paper,' continues the Poetess, obliviously, 'I have written:

> "Give me a corner of your heart,
> That I may fill with memories,
> To fill your dreams
> Forever."

I am embarking on a study of the concept of randomness in poetry. What is your opinion?'

'No one in Mongolia could possibly have thought of that,' say I. 'Surely not?'

Content, the Hungry Poetess descends the stairs to fulfil her appointment with the Doctor.

We hurry to the now over-familiar Jorge Chávez Airport, with thoughts of heroic pioneering flights over the Alps uppermost in our minds. La Señora is evident from afar, wearing reindeer boots and trundling her trolley, the universal leveller. She departed with three suitcases, now there are four.

'Wait,' says the Doctor, 'something is left.'

He is right. Another large suitcase is added to the baggage cart. I knew she would not disappoint us.

'These are my luggages,' explains the returning traveller.

La Señora is tired. 'Jet flag' she calls it. Not to mention all those dinner parties, all those ice cubes.

'On the long flight I did my book. I did my nail polish. Then it was time to do something else. "Where are you from?" I ask my neighbour. "Do you care too much?" he retorts. So I tell the stewardess to move me to another seat and she does. Now I am a shrunk person,' declares La Señora. 'In Europe everyone is shrunk. It is the weather.'

She is not going to be rushed into relating the epic story of her odyssey to the whitely frozen wastes.

'I need to be relax.'

We wait patiently for the next pronouncement.

'If you go to a place you don't know,' she informs us, 'you are out of your knowledge.' There is a pause. 'When you move from one place to another, you lose the string.'

Silence, whilst we reflect on this, followed by a further declaration.

'Carefully listen. Snow is the rain of the angels. Before, no one gave value to this activity.'

Snow or ice sculpture? La Señora is warming the audience.

She tells how she herself was granted an audience with Father Christmas and how she visited an ice bar in an ice hotel. Tables and chairs all in ice, even the instruments for the orchestra. Really? Suddenly comes a revelation.

'The Japaneezee Hashi Moto finished his carving in one day.'

Brother of Mickey? Anyway, bad form. The judges notice things like that. Lack of effort.

'The Korean complained about the size of his block. He said, "I don't like this block."'

Well, he would, wouldn't he? North or South? In ice, when the chips are down, it's volume that counts. Size matters.

'The Korean was ten centimetres short,' continues La Señora.

My goodness! That's a lot!

'What happened next?' we ask.

They gave him a new block with the yellow machine.'

'The yellow machine?'

'Yes, the ice tractor. Then he won.'

'¡*Miércoles!* Ten centimetres short and he won!'

'On the bottom of his new block he wrote "Open the mind". It was a message to the judges.'

'*Miércoles* again!' Open the mind? Make a note of that for next time.

'What about Eric, the one in the photograph?'

'He was a pastry chef. Ice is different to icing. There was also a Swedish chef. This man here in the picture is a Swedish. It was Eric against the Swedish pastry.'

'And the Serbs? What happened to Serbia?'

'On the day, they were not inspired. In fact they were spaced out and *pensativo*. This Serb is only smiling because he has new teeth.'

We look closely at the photographs.

'I didn't take enough presents. Just llamas and *las zampoñas*, the mountain pipes. In the end my new friends were looking to my eyes to see what else I could give them. I just told them

181

"My heart is overflowing with milk and honey, but sadly my hands are empty". Of course they laughed, but not with happiness.'

Wonderful. 'Would you like to hear our news? We are all tiptop and the Clinic is quite fine too.' No need to elaborate with unnecessary, inconsequential details.

'Who? What?'

'You know, Dr Desastre and everyone, all fine. Dr Ching comes and goes and Dr Vonday is still with us. The garden is flourishing but we were just wondering if we might sell a few things, maybe a few cars and a bit of land, so we can pay back the Bank a little. Then perhaps we could even install the lift to move the patients upstairs? After deliveries . . . '

Silence. Our eyes fall to the floor.

'Possibly we could sell the plant nursery at Huachipa, you know, that kind of thing, no one goes there any more, or even some of the farm, or something . . . ?'

Silence. We look up. La Señora has left. The silence of space.

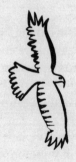

16

Peruvian Peregrinations

For our sporadic weekly staff meetings, held monthly, La Señora dons the white linen coat that habitually hangs unmolested on the hook behind her office door. Thus attired, and as we glaze and glide through the latest performance statistics, and Nurse Dulce, Ernestina and Señorita Hilda receive exhortations in triplicate concerning the length of their occasionally delightfully indecorous skirts, the regrettable advisability of bun-tight hair arrangements in preference to wildly suggestive flamenco tresses, punctilious observance of the hour and the absolute avoidance of the colour black in their wardrobes, the proceedings are graced with an appropriate clinical ambience.

At the gathering following her return from the Ice, the Headmistress unusually bids me stay behind as the others troop from the auditorium to recover their shoes lined up by the door.

'To cure your stress,' declares La Señora, dispensing with preliminaries, 'I have decided that you shall travel. It will be a *bendición* for you.'

'Stress?'

'Do not tire yourself by speaking,' comes the swift admonition. 'I have diagnosed that you are enduring severe emotional disturbance resulting from serious overwork during my absence.'

'Golly!' Suddenly that white coat has assumed new significance.

'The proposal to part with my plant nursery at Huachipa has left me furruffled and I will therefore companion you to Cusco and to Machu Picchu. They are places with very much age,' she adds thoughtfully, looking at me as though I might have had a hand in their construction.

So it is that quite soon afterwards at 4.30 in the morning there we are again at Jorge Chávez Airport, the fragile fortunes of the Clinic once more entrusted to the loyal surrogates. We are in the company of the world and his llama, also flying to Cusco and also wishing they were still in bed. The real truth of the matter is that La Señora, when not engaged on international artistic commitments, is a devoted traveller. So we negotiate the congested check-in circuit, close to chaos, we say 'no thank you' to the whispered offer from one official to change our tickets to those of another airline in return for a ten-dollar bonus and finally we take our allotted seats.

Arriving at our destination, I attend to the baggage and lose La Señora. The Cusco altitude of 11,000 feet is not to her liking, in spite of her childhood at the family hacienda near Puno. She is located in the first-aid post, relaxing on a couch and sipping oxygen through a mask. If she could have imbibed the elixir from a glass with a long stem she would have been even more contented on the chaise-longue.

La Señora looks at me curiously from the comfort of her pillow, bent as I am under the weight of her suitcases.

'Are you tired?' she enquires. 'I don't wish to be a kind of bothering person, but you are breathing strangely. Before I see you very well in good shape. For your age, that is, and apart from the overwork. But now what is happening in your mind? Well, you may rest if that's what you want. It is true, here we are well more than three thousand metres tall.'

She lies back on her pillows, breathes deeply, exhausts the gas cylinder without soliciting my assistance and feels better, ready to marvel at the architectural wonders of Cusco, Inca capital and 'navel of the world' in the Quechua language; the 'dwelling place of the gods' founded by Manco Capac and Mama Ocllo, the legendary original Incas who sprang from the waters of Lake Titicaca. Many of the early buildings with their distinctive, intricately interlocking stonework were destroyed by the invading Spanish; in turn many of the Spanish buildings, some constructed from the Inca stones, were demolished or damaged in subsequent earthquakes.

We move onward to explore the Sacsayhuaman military fortress, then to picturesque Pisac ('These house walls are adobe, just mud, not so many other condiments'), through the Sacred Valley of Urubamba to equally harmonious Ollantaytambo ('From the cross on the roof of these old houses you see two bottles; one for the holy water and one for the liquor to be happy in the home'). We reach the lost citadel of Machu Picchu by taking the rattling single-track train to the mountaintop, economically deny ourselves a return by helicopter and regret it for ever after.

La Señora then decrees that we should fly directly south from Cusco to the 'white city' of Arequipa, *ciudad natal* for Dr Hermogenes, *la tierra del Misti*, land of Misti, the majestic volcano, where references to the 'Republic of Arequipa' are made only half in jest. Amidst family lunches and dinners we visit the cathedral in the Plaza de Armas, we walk through the Convent of Santa Catalina, over 400 years old ('So much here is from the early days'), we see the sadly contorted remains of 'Juanita', Ice Maiden of Ampato, the 14-year-old Inca girl sacrificed 500 years previously, and to restore our energy after journeying so far through time, we cross Gustave Eiffel's Puente de Hierro, using his narrow iron bridge over *el río* Chili to visit the family *anís* factory and to drink fortifying pisco sours at the Libertador Plaza Hotel.

Revitalized we go to La Casa del Fundador, the restored hacienda of the city's founder. As we are engaged in admiring the treasures of the chapel, a vivid magenta geranium diverts our attention. The necessary cuttings are being taken for propagation in the Clinic garden when, quite unannounced, Mother Superior appears on the terrace. La Señora, forever equal to the moment, pops the plant pieces down the front of her dress, smiles innocently and the time of day is passed pleasantly with *la madre superiora*. Happily, there are no bolts of lightning and later La Señora ('You placed me in a very ashamed situation') sets about recovering the stems from the secret depths of her person. They have sunk further than anticipated, no doubt on account of gravity and curiosity in equal measure. La Señora is forced to retire but soon returns successfully waving aloft the slightly squashed and bruised bundle of warm cuttings.

'They'll be fine,' she pronounces, but I am not so sanguine. A few weeks later when they have all died, in spite of the utmost horticultural efforts, I seek a medical opinion from the Doctor as to why such an unfortunate thing should have occurred. He is unhesitating and unequivocal.

'Trauma,' he declares. 'A severe case of cataleptic shock.' He should know.

The weeks pass. Clinical business is transacted much as before: the patients come and go, Señorita Hilda, Ernestina and Nurse Dulce flit to and fro, the doctors preside with white-coated professional calm. Stressful and furruffling mention of asset sales is assiduously avoided, notwithstanding the fact that with patient numbers static, and imagined essential expenditures equally immovable, the obvious route to financial salvation is loan interest reduction. On occasions, cash-flow mishaps lead to non-payment of the telephone bills, whereupon Telefónica takes swift revenge and cuts the lines. At first, La Señora perceives this as an excellent economy curb but after a day or two with ever-dwindling appointments, reason prevails and contact with the outside world is resumed.

Meantime, the presidential election is drawing closer, and with it the faint hope of economic changes. The small matter of the one million additional voting signatures remains unresolved. No, says the relevant government department, we cannot possibly look into the situation prior to the election. You must understand how busy we are at this moment. We cannot be expected to conduct an investigation and an election simultaneously, whatever next? And by the way, you should be aware that the reporter responsible for bringing this alleged episode to light just happens to be a thief, a drug addict, a homosexual and a murderer. Simultaneously, *El Comercio*, valiant purveyor of unwelcome news, falls prey to sinister and subtle pressures. The freedom of the press is at stake. An overseas observer and political analyst, writing from a safe distance, declares that a 'slow-motion' coup d'état is in process in Peru. The only thing that remains constant is invisible Ezequiel, with his popularity steadfast at half of one per cent.

Against this backdrop, the discovery that distribution of aid from a major foreign charitable programme is being accompanied by presidential electioneering propaganda barely makes the front page of the dailies. Then the Government raises the national minimum wage by twenty per cent. Do not be confused, the President assures, this is not an electioneering ploy.

Unconnected, we receive an invitation from the Minister of

Health, keen to integrate the private, charitable and public health sectors, to go north to visit hospitals and *postas medicas* and simultaneously to view the devastation wrought by El Niño, the wilful consequence of that periodic aberration occurring in the normally cool waters of the Humboldt Current. We fly to tropical Tumbes, unexcitable, amiable and architecturally undistinguished, from where in 1527 Francisco Pizarro sallied forth to defeat the Incas, and from where we visit the border with Ecuador at the frontier township of Aguas Verdes before driving south down the coast, breaking the journey at the beaches of Punta Sal and Mancora to ride horses along the deserted sands.

'I need to be near the ocean,' says La Señora, 'I am like that. Maybe I was born in the ocean, *una sirena*, a mermaid. Or maybe I was only a tiny grain of sand on the edge of the great waters. Here every day is a shiny sun day. Now these eyes are happy, they are seeing different vistas.'

Talking of which, the minuscule bikini that La Señora has selected from her extensive collection as the sartorial topping for her equestrian excursion proves to be unequal to the challenging torques and torsions presented by a rollicking canter, whereupon our guide, clearly a competent horseman in normal circumstances, practically falls from his mount at the heaven-sent vision of Lady Godiva that has unexpectedly appeared at his elbow.

Order restored, further along the beach we encounter an ancient crone, wizened beyond belief, bent double and tottering under the weight of her load of diurnal driftwood for the kitchen fire. Overcome with compassion, La Señora's soft-hearted, moist-eyed reaction is immediate: the charitable aims of our satellite clinics for the poor and needy shall be extended forthwith to include the provision of donkeys for all such persons, wherever they may be, and please kindly remind her of this on return to the office. So be it; no point in speculating at this stage exactly how many driftwood donkeys might be required.

188

Then we sample crabs and lobsters within sight of the timeless waves, those sinuous rolling visitors from far-off Tahiti, garlanded with spindrift, surf and spray.

'The seafood comes from only there to here. It is not fair not to eat it,' explains my companion. 'Along our coast we have many little islands and I have learnt that on these islands are many little snails. You feed them scallops and they flavour scallops; you feed them crabs and they taste crabs. One day soon I shall do this and I will be rich again.'

Onward with the Minister we travel the Pan Americana highway, swept away in parts by the El Niño rains, past the 'nodding donkeys' in the oilfields of Talara and through the rice fields of Sullana, to arrive in gentle Piura, with its *algarrobo* trees and fine university, long after nightfall. From the *algarrobo* or carob tree comes the health-giving *algarrobina* syrup, but before we can partake of the assorted minerals, proteins and vitamins of the renowned potion for *impotencia*, it is the Piura Bridge, or more accurately the late Piura Bridge, that is forced upon our attention. The dust of travel hardly shaken from our clothes, we learn from concerned citizens that this vital city link over the River Piura had been destroyed by the raging El Niño flood waters just two years previously. Furthermore, we are told, this British-constructed bridge had lasted since 1893, having been diverted or hijacked at the penultimate hour from its originally intended destination in India. Subsequent to the inconvenient and dramatic demise of the Anglo-Indian bridge, an unnamed Chinaman with a previous history of engineering misfortune had been engaged to build a replacement. Unfortunately his bad luck held and his ill-fated effort toppled into the fast-flowing waters of the river scarcely before the bolts had been tightened and with the paint hardly dry. We listen to the sorry tale with polite interest, deliberately declining in any way to relate the circumstances to our arrival in town.

However, given the narrated history of the broken bridges,

given the arrival of La Señora's mythical British Lord, what happens next is predictable. After all, a request for one new bridge once every hundred years is hardly exorbitant. We undertake to look into the matter with the British Embassy, urgently, and our word is our bond, even though the hidden undercurrents of La Señora's creative marketing have unexpectedly swept us on to uncharted shoals. Nevertheless, before hastening back to Lima we make time to go shopping in the old town of Catacaos, close by Piura and home of the *toquilla* straw hats much favoured by the builders of the Panama Canal, hence the subsequent misnomer.

Tappity-tap, tappity-tap, familiar mid-morning feet excitedly climbing the fourth-floor stairs.

'¡*Oye!* Listen!' exclaims La Señora still ascending – so imperiously that the startled pigeons in the dead tree suffer communal coitus interruptus and scatter for their lives in fluttering fear. I swivel calmly in my senior management chair to await events; this is not the first such commotion to be encountered hereabouts.

'¡*Oye!*' says La Señora once again and now ascended, just to ensure that my attention is undivided. 'Here's what we must do.' I watch the pigeons circling out of the corner of my eye. 'Our patient numbers are limited in this moment by the economical conditions. Also, and as you know, I have drastically dropped our regular expenditures. So, what remains?' Dramatic pause. The pigeons are wondering if it is safe to return to the dead tree. 'The loan! We must reduce the money we owe to the Bank! Then we can pay less interest and all will be saved!' At the crescendo of this denouement the pigeons take fright again.

'*¡Dios mío!*' It is inadequate to the moment, but it is the best I can manage.

'So,' concludes La Señora, 'that's what we will do and we may start today.'

However, the political uncertainties in Peru are an impediment to our refinancing efforts for the Clinic. If only we could reduce the overdraft interest rate to sensible single figures then all would be well. We could go the races, decorate the consulting rooms with endless bulls, spend unworried weeks at the beach, travel endlessly and fill the shelves of the medical library with learned tomes. We could even buy the vital lift to move patients from downstairs delivery to their rooms on the third floor.

We try bank after bank, but to no avail.

'This is not a game of throwing and pulling,' La Señora tells the grey men. 'This is not the ceremony of the tea. I do not wish all my eggs to be in the one nest. See for this, we need to work with less interest, otherwise you are killing us. Be knowing that if you sharpen the pencil too much, the pencil gets small. The monies that are due now I wish to pass them to the back. You need to forgive the payments for a while, that will be fine. You may be sure that in time I will pay my debts with noble-ty but at this moment you are taking the chocolates without the hunger, just the greed.'

Such innovations are beyond the scope of the grey men. We write letters; we do not receive the courtesy of a response.

'I am discontent, my mind is upset,' says La Señora. 'It is life to be in dispute but they must reply me.' But they don't. It is the way. La Señora is disconsolate. 'I feel I have no future,' she says. 'I am flattened like a frog in a high way.'

'On a highway,' I amend.

'Yes, a flat frog on a high way,' she accepts impatiently. 'I must be calmed down and learn to grow old gracefully. I need someone with me in the end of my winter, with the sprinkle of snow in my hair, to help me in my ancient times. That person

191

Luzmila was right, to hold my hand and to tight the fingers very much.'

In war, love and oratory, moderation is madness.

As a last resort, we approach an old friend of La Señora's, now a senior financier. Poor chap, he is suffering from a serious excess of gravitas. No jokes from him over the kippers.

'He is too much a calmed down person,' says La Señora. 'In fact he is a boring to death person. I met his wife. She was a French. Of course, you know that to save moments that's why the French are not using the underclothes? Anyway, now she is gone. This man, he was my first boyfriend and he tried to hold my hand. It was a violation. Such an insult to touch the body. Of course, I spanked him in the face.'

At this revelation I sense the return of that familiar no-bigger-than-a-man's-hand cloud on the distant horizon. Nevertheless, a meeting is arranged and La Señora explains our predicament.

'I am telling you everything,' she says to the gloomy money man. 'I am putting all the dishes on the table. To the banks I confess them all my problems, even though they treat me like a miserable. These people are laughing out of me. I want to smile and be happy. With the Clinic, I put my best on it. I am a very good entertainment person, always joking and jumping but still I am a good worker. Believe me, I am a serious person too. I am telling you this because I know that in business you can only give the money to the people you can trust on. Now you have the handle of the pan in your hand.'

Notwithstanding the rhetoric, the old boyfriend with the new money regrets that he is unable to help us. Maybe he has a long memory. Or merely those oft-found short arms, deep pockets and no vision. In fact, the longer we brood about it, the more obvious it becomes that he is the sort of mega-mean person who can sur-reptitiously peel an orange in his pocket and spirit the segments to his mouth by sleight of hand to obviate the pulverizing pos-sibility of having to share a single section, even one slippery pip.

192

'This person put down my day,' observes La Señora. 'He just says "no" and quite unnecessarily he repeated it twice. For him to smile is expensive; for me it is free. For him a smile is a sign of weakness. A "thank you" is an unacceptable burden of debt. His moods are from the mountains. Darkly foreboding, gloom-full, what is the word? Why is he talking stupidities?'

'Saturnine.' I wait for the finale and I am duly rewarded.

'All right. Don't think that he will long last saturnine more than six months. He is very fat. He cannot make love, he cannot do nothing. His colleagues they don't like him, he is always foolishing them. He's finished, soon he will die flat. In fact, he is already dead. Just the two feet are walking. Sorry for that but I cannot keep my words.'

We retreat from the congested centre of Lima, where the pollution levels comfortably exceed all known criteria for at least 365 days every year and return disconsolately to the haven of the Clinic in Miraflores. Without the need for questions, Señorita Hilda puts the kettle on to prepare fortifying motherly mugs of *maté de coca*, Nurse Dulce drops her doleful eyes and Ernestina scuttles to safety, seeking refuge under the stairs.

'Whenever I have a disagreeable with the banks,' says La Señora, staring at the waterless water feature unseeingly from her glass-fronted office adjacent to the auditorium, 'I pray and I cry. Here I send you the tears of the ocean. Too distracted am I. My eyes they cry alone. I cannot cry any more. I have never seen a person cry so much as me, my tears they splash to my hands, my face it runs to the floor. My tears are like golden grapes, it is too expensive. In life, the heart must be as an open flower, welcoming to the inquisitive butterflies. I make too many prays, I think. God is not listening.'

'Those sowing seed with tears,' I quote prophetically, 'shall reap and harvest even with a joyful cry.' But now it is La Señora who is not listening.

'At this time, I am the one suffering from stress, if not from overwork,' she continues. 'How sad it is to pass by the world without stepping in every corner.' La Señora is restless. 'We need to move around in this life. It may take me a long time to get to China but I will do it. Of course, and as you may know, I will need to learn how to walk in the rain because I never had such a thing, but yes, I can do it. Let us go and seek the harmony of happiness or happiness in harmony. Lima is too heavy for us, now we must leave.'

Day by day, the prospect of taking the keys of the Clinic to the Bank is increasingly becoming a reality. 'Here,' we shall say. 'Take them. Take your pound of flesh. We have done our best. You have done your worst. Do what you like with our beautiful dream. We have other things to do with our lives. We are here for but a short time and, as far as we know, we are here only once. Life is once, *sí o no*?'

Everything indicates that the time has indeed come for a little more recuperative travelling.

'Why don't we go to tranquil Tarma?' say I, over lunch in Casa Bonomini. 'My book says that it is the Pearl of the Andes and City of Flowers, where, after braving the snow-covered peaks of the Anticona Pass, we may be embraced at ten thousand feet by the eccentric hospitality of Hotel Los Portales with bizarre plumbing and a blazing fire of eucalyptus logs and tour the terraced flower fields filled with industrious *campesinos* tending gladioli, gypsophila, carnations, stocks and statice. And spinach. Then, encouraged by this glimpse of paradise, we may travel through the sweetly scented orange and tangerine plantations of the Chanchamayo Valley, one-time territory of the native Asháninka people.'

La Señora reaches over the salt and pepper and takes the guide book. 'It says we could also go to Huaraz,' she paraphrases, 'not-to-be-missed access point for the spectacular Cordillera Blanca where we may walk on the ice of Glacier Pastoruri, soon to be obliterated by global warming, before visiting the memorial gardens of Yungay where eighty thousand people, *eighty thousand*, were eradicated in mud in 1970. Also in this section is Huancayo, two hundred kilometres east of Lima, in the scenically fertile Mantaro Valley where the presidential decree abolishing slavery in Peru was signed in 1854. Population: one quarter of a million people surrounded by *retama*, the yellow flowering broom. I have not before been that way.'

'You should go by train,' advises knowledgeable Dr Hermogenes. 'It is the highest railway in the world, called "the railway to the moon", 15,688 feet at Ticlio, built by Henry Meiggs who should have been an Englishman but wasn't. He had a vision to "scale the summits of the Andes and to unite with bonds of iron the people of the Pacific and the Atlantic". He ran out of money.'

'From the mountains of Peru you may kiss the sky, you may feel "the high untrespassed sanctity of space and put out your hand to touch the face of God",' misquotes La Señora, not to be left out.

'The fare is thirty nuevos soles, less than ten dollars, lunch and oxygen included, for a twelve-hour ride,' continues the Doctor. 'That is the going. I don't know about the coming back. Maybe in a box,' he concludes happily.

'Have you ever felt how hot your bottom comes when you sit too much?' enquires La Señora, of no one in particular, and then further consults the guide book, finally breaking the silence to announce her decision. 'We shall go north to Cajamarca, the Little Switzerland of Peru.' She closes the book and lays it on the table.

Undeterred, the Doctor simulates a further reading. 'Cajamarca,' he intones, 'land of the lustful locusts, devouring all before them, pausing only to indulge in twenty-four-hour bouts of heroic non-stop fornication.'

'We are in a time of economy,' observes La Señora, ignoring such puerile comments. 'You put me the ticket for the plane and then you come in the bus.'

But it is over 800 kilometres, a long day on the road, studying at first hand how it is that the motor coaches of Peru crash with such regularity, tumbling into rivers and ravines at an average of one a week. It will be through no fault of our driver's if we chance to arrive at our destination safely, using the horn in preference to the brakes, accelerating towards any hint of danger to demonstrate a clear sense of purpose. I have a better idea. Air tickets for everyone, even though the flight leaves before dawn.

'It is very early,' sighs La Señora. 'To get up this early is a crime. At the early morning I could not wish to wake up.'

In the historic city of Cajamarca is El Cuarto del Rescate, the Ransom Room that the captured Inca Chief Atahualpa filled with gold to the height of his fingertips to buy his freedom from Francisco Pizarro in 1532. Only to be garrotted anyway by the perfidious pig farmer just nine months later. Further afield are Las Ventanillas de Otuzco, the macabre 'hanging tombs' with bodies lodged in burial holes carved in the cliff face; then we go high into the mountain pine forests, the green valleys dotted with dairy herds far below, where the concepts of the infinite and the eternal become realities.

'For the size of the country,' La Señora tells me, 'we do not have so many people.'

With much to see, I forget the banalities of life and omit to reconfirm our return flight.

'How could you do such a thing?' exclaims La Señora.

Oh, quite easily, really.

At the hotel I am ostracized by my fellow travellers, banished to the far end of the thermal pool with only the bubbling hot springs for company. In an effort to reingratiate myself, I hold secret consultations with the receptionist who makes some unpromising-sounding telephone calls on my behalf.

'These expenses are improving your bill, heh?' observes La Señora, mirthfully and uncharitably, as she unexpectedly catches me in my sotto voce endeavours.

'It should be all right,' the receptionist tells me, as we both pretend to be alone at the desk. Definitely unpromising. Peruvians never say 'no'. Except for the banks. It is far too brutal. It is not what the listener wants to hear. 'Yes' means 'maybe'. Anything else means, 'no way, José'. Grammatically, to spare the speaker the crippling embarrassment of having to say 'no', Castellano offers no fewer than six assorted variants of the elusive *subjuntivo*, and umpteen other linguistic devices. The humble visitor need not be master of these subtle techniques; sufficient to know of their existence, thereby saving a deal of disappointment. Who coined the phrase 'a Peruvian promise'? Anonymous, but surely the voice of experience.

It's all about adjusting to the rhythm and music of the language, attuning to the cadence of the country, the personality of Peru. To have a second language is indeed 'to have a second soul'. Just as 'no' is simply too inconceivably negative to countenance, 'yes' is similarly too incredibly positive. In consequence, 'maybe', 'hopefully' and 'possibly' feature frequently in Peruvian conversations. No one has the faintest idea who is doing what and when and to whom, but nobody cares and that's not the point. Only Europeans, North Americans and a handful of others still cling to the convention that from time to time conversations should possibly relate to an exchange of definite information.

I report back to the group. They are still in the hotel pool, relaxing happily in the renowned therapeutic thermal waters.

'It should be all right!' I tell them.

The laughter and the chatter cease. The pariah is at the pool-side. The one who forgot to reconfirm the flights.

'I am not sure about all these "all rights",' comments that well-known voice. 'I do not think they are all right at all. Nothing happens all right to me.'

We move to the airport.

'It should be all right,' says the check-in girl. 'Hopefully.' *Ojalá*, always followed by the *subjuntivo*, the big let out.

The group ignore me, so I whistle a happy tune and go outside to take advantage of the scenery and the fresh, fresh air of Cajamarca. There is a high wooden platform on one side of the runway, which must be the control tower. Underneath the structure is a man with a pair of binoculars slung round his neck, who must be the air traffic controller. He gazes at the sky periodically with his glasses, in between throwing sticks for his dog to retrieve. All at once his radio crackles.

'Cajamarca, Cajamarca,' says a voice from the clouds. Pilots and people like that always say things twice. 'Come in Cajamarca. Come in Cajamarca.'

'Here boy! Here boy!' says ground control.

'Say again, Cajamarca. Say again.'

'Good dog, Neron! Good dog!'

'We have interference, we have interference,' crackle the clouds. 'Report your weather, your weather.'

'We are quite fine here, quite fine,' reports ground control, scaling the scaffolding to reach the platform and scanning the clouds for the mystery voice, whilst Neron pants patiently at the foot of the ladder, stick in mouth.

Suddenly the scheduled Fokker-Whatever appears over the peaks and makes a thundering low pass down the runway. Air Traffic Control follows the aircraft's progress with his binoculars. It must be all of fifty metres distant. Neron yelps and takes cover behind the platform.

The conditions are not to the pilot's liking.

'*Adiós*, Cajamarca, *adiós*.' Crackle, crackle. Even the radio repeats itself. '*Hasta mañana*, see you tomorrow.'

The crosswind may have been quite fine for Neron and his twigs, but it's quite another thing for a Fokker-Whatever. So that's it then. *Adiós* to you too. With a waggle of his wings the pilot heads for home and a nice cup of tea with his wife and I head back to the departure lounge. Ground Control shrugs and lowers his binoculars. *Mañana*.

'Here boy! Here boy!'

With a wag of his tail Neron is ready for the next stick.

I go to see the check-in girl, now at the check-out desk.

'Señorita,' I say, as my Castellano enjoys a rare moment of fluency, 'I wonder if we could reconfirm our flights for tomorrow, please?'

'Yes, that should be all right,' she tells me.

I give the glad news to the group as we drive back to the hotel for another night in the thermal pool.

'She says it should be all right!'

I really want to tell everyone that, after all, it didn't matter that I forgot to reconfirm the flights. It was the weather, see? Tricky katabatic crosswind for the Fokker. But in life it's not the truth which matters. It's what people believe that counts. So nobody talks to me and nobody comes to my end of the pool. It's nothing really. I don't care.

A few days later when we are back in Lima, La Señora unexpectedly turns to me.

'You remember at Cajamarca that happy dog with the stick? Neron, *sí*? I had a dog once. His name was Spottie. Oh, we were so good friends. We were so close all day long, and at night Spottie was under my bed for company. I also had a mad uncle.

One day, soon after my father had died, this uncle came to me and said, "Say goodbye to your dog now." And I remember my dog looking to me with his eyes. And my mad uncle shot my dog. I was four years old. I never spoke to him again. My father was killed in a crash. He was the finest flyer in all the air force, but the engine of his plane stopped and he fell to the mountains. He was thirty-three and I was four. I couldn't have the age to help that feather fly again. I believed that he went to the paradise to visit God and that he would soon be back. I wait many years to see him back. One day, maybe soon, he will come and hold my hand and take me with him and then we can fly together, as he always promised, like two feathers all over the skies. I will not forget my brushes and I will paint the stars high above the clouds and of course I will put a little bit of sparkling dust to surround them in the darkness. Maybe you will be one of them and I promise to visit you and give you a nice kiss and your face will turn red and maybe you will want to follow us, my father and me.'

Just three days absent from the capital, plus the extra one as things turned out, now to catch up with events. The tempo of the presidential election is accelerating. Exciting news, 'El Cholo', the contender from the mountains, is closing on 'El Chino', presidential incumbent and paradoxically from Japan. For the no-hopers down the line, little change. Octogenarian candidate Ezequiel is still showing excellent consistency with his half per cent scoop of the electorate, whereas for the mounted candidate who has opted to run his forgettable campaign from the saddle there is double disappointment. Polls reveal that the voters prefer the horse to the rider and that he is unrecognizable without his mount. Like his Wild West hat, he needs to wear the horse inside and out. By way of consolation the dastardly rumour is put about that the horse is gay.

More depressingly for the weary candidates, all their efforts are anyway to no avail: surveys show that one third of the electorate are unclear how to complete the newly introduced ballot forms and many of the votes will be nullified. Surely it can't be that complicated? Only if you want it to be. For one thing, the void will leave ample room should anyone wish to add, say, one million fraudulent votes to the electoral roll. A national magazine gives a reminder that in the elections five years previously, less than half of the nine million votes were adjudged valid and more than four million votes effectively disappeared. Any advance on that will be progress.

Simultaneously squinting on the future and the present, we investigate another source of funding for the Clinic, a personal contact. The answer is the same. Always the same.

'Once upon a time, this man he was the most richest man in all Peru,' explains La Señora. 'He is very known here, but now, unfortunately, maybe he is not too well in money. It seems that the money has been going out. In fact, he is empty of money, one hand here, one hand in the back. He is so low on the gravity that he is decreasing very fast.'

So much for that. We know all about this business of the money going out. We need to seek salvation elsewhere and I spend long hours gazing dreamily at the pigeons in the dead tree. Apparently, pigeons have difficulty in focusing properly. I learnt this from Medical Student One, who read it in a book of his. That's why they move their heads back and forth when they walk. I watch intently. There! Forward go the heads to see where they are going, back again to see where they are, or maybe where they have been. Amazing. Forward, back. Forward, back. I reach out to ring Medical Student One at Casa Bonomini with my findings, only to discover that the lines are down again.

'LEAVE LIMA IMMEDIATELY!'

My barren inspirational reverie disintegrates in an explosion of cascading colour like a dropped kaleidoscope and I jump violently in my swivelling senior management desk chair.

'*¿Perdón?*' No warning tappity-tap on the stairs today. The enemy has adopted the latest stealth techniques to tiptoe through my early warning defences.

'The woman with the broken muffler has been here, *sí o no*?' La Señora glares at the sheet of verse that she is brandishing. Is nothing sacred?

'*¿Perdón?* The Hungry Poetess? Well, *sí*, it's true. How can I stop people coming up these stairs? It happens all the time. Anyway, I don't even know her name, but she's lonely. There's no need to get furruffled.'

'It's very astonishing. "The Song of the Surf Gatherers"? What is this concoction?'

'I quite like it,' I protest feebly. Then she starts to read in a quirkily amazed voice.

'"The sand gilt shore stretched straight before
   Way beyond and as far could be
And along the sand the rollers ran
   Ran rolling from the sea.

The sun shone bright as the sand shone white
   And the sky sat still on the earth
But along the shore the rollers wore
   Their racing caps of surf.

And as they rolled on the sand of gold
   The spindrift danced with mirth
Whilst from the land came another band
   Came the men that gathered surf.

And as this band played on the sand
   And the rollers raced along

The surfmen sung as the surf they wrung
  And these were the sings of their song."

'I cannot go on,' sighs La Señora, a living portrait of personified exasperation. 'There are six more such verses. There must
be a deeply hidden significance here. I knew I had put too
many flowers on your head. We cannot risk losing you. You
belong to The Ladies' Healthcare Clinic, Lima.'

'The point is,' I offer, by way of placatory clarification, 'the
surf makes patterns in the sand, which can be read like a chart,
symbolistic of future journeys.' The grammatical lapse betrays
my remorse.

La smouldering Señora turns on her expensively shod heel
and departs in a reverberating silence. The ultimate sanction.

Two minutes later she is back.

'You will enjoy the Amazon,' she declares, in a conciliatory
tone. 'I am not myself for *la selva*, I am not for the adventure of
the forest. The boas and the anacondas are not to my liking. In
the jungle there are no stars. Just the darkness of the trees
pressing down like a prison. That is not good for my soul,
alone except for the quiet rustling of the leaves praising the
heavens. No, I am not a bird of the forest in the cages of the
trees; I am a bird of *la costa*, a free spirit of the ocean. And generally I am more for the *jungla cemento*. But I fix your going.
Immediately. You are going out from Lima, that's important.
You looks like a happy man; maybe you are a man from the
jungle or for the jungle. You go beautiful and you will have
total relax. There they often sleep in hamcocks. When you
arrive you can get together with some friends and then you are
not extremely alone. Have a nice time in the jungles but be
careful please, in *la selva* they might put you to boil in a
pot, totally uncondimented. And avoid eating snakes and
monkey's brains, they can have a curious effect on a person.
And remember you may only eat or drink those things that you

see prepared before your eyes. My mother taught me never to drink anything from other hands. For some people the jungle and the coconuts are getting them crazy and they never return. Many people they put money in the jungle and they lost; the jungle didn't give the body.'

It is true that wildlife and La Señora have some degree of incompatibility. Not long ago a spider crossed her kneecap and she was rushed to hospital for emergency treatment. The whole event turned into a fiesta. Word of the drama spread like a pampas blaze and in no time La Señora's ward was filled with a crush of concerned supporters, so that the grave ministrations of the medical staff became completely inaudible over the fizz of the party, the clink of glasses and the noise of chatter and popping corks. Private healthcare is a wonderful thing. Except, of course, the cost.

As for the boas and anacondas, well, I too have reservations on that score. Not that South America, hairy-chested continent of the unbuttoned shirt and gold medallion, is the place to admit such pathetic phobias. And La Señora's offer to make the travel arrangements? Marvellous.

For me, travel agencies reserve a de luxe line in rejections. First I try the telephone, in Peru not always the most rewarding part of the day. Then I visit personally, which is the signal for the entire agency staff to glare fixedly at their computers, where they are undoubtedly playing Patience or Pokémon. I shuffle up and down the counter hopefully. Nobody moves.

'Have a chair,' suggests the receptionist, a good-hearted, big-breasted girl, unsettled by my pacing.

Fatal. Sit down and you become part of the scenery, someone with time to lose, someone to be ignored. So I continue my shuffling, to and fro, imagining that the generous-seeming receptionist must be called Abundancia, although I can't be certain because she doesn't tell me. For the Pokémon players my pacing is like the water torture. Drip, drip, drip. Finally I win. A bad-tempered girl, probably named Nina Carwanka, looks up from her grumpy screen.

'You want something?' she snaps. The scowling moon face is longer than the question.

'One fillet steak, please. Medium rare.' Sometimes I am the author of my own misfortunes. 'And a nice bottle of red wine.'

'Sorry?'

'I need to travel. Immediately.'

'Name?' What's that got to do with it? But I tell her anyway.

'Can you spell that?'

'Of course I can.' What is this, an IQ test?

'Do you have a ticket?'

'No, for goodness' sake, that's why I'm here.'

'All right! All right! I'm only asking!'

'OK! OK! I'm only telling you!'

Oh dear. Yes, it would be most helpful if La Señora could make the arrangements for the jungle journey. Meantime, I recall reading previously in the guide book about Amazonia. From memory, it said: '*La selva* is reputedly peopled by warm women of serpentine form, as exquisite as the orchids of the woodland, fresh and crisp as lettuces sparkling in the early morning dew, where the midnight maidens of the forest dance naked in vibrant fertility rites, circling fruit-laden mango and *mamey* trees with the faint rays of the new moon, the silent witness, caressing their glistening gluteus'. I wonder if La Señora is privy to this information, or whether perhaps my memory has been affected by the inspirational pigeon-laden dead tree. Either way, and overreaction or not, I resolve to accept my temporary banishment with good grace.

Thus it is that I arrive in the happy city of Iquitos, hot and humid, frontier outpost of the Peruvian rainforest. To my surprise and as in Arequipa, *ingeniero* Gustave Eiffel has again beaten me to it. So I stop for dinner in La Casa de Fierro and, on the balcony of the iron house designed by the French architect, consume an alligator steak, surreally served by a deaf waiter bereft of teeth.

The following day I drift downstream on the mighty 'monarch of the rivers', and disappear. From under the blanket of clouds and sheets of rain over the womb of my bed I listen that night to *la sinfonía de la selva* before taking a canoe on the misty waters of the Amazon. As artfully intended by La Señora, Lima has been left far behind. Except that, with astonishment that must have equalled that of Dr Livingstone and Mr Stanley in another jungle in another age, I chance to meet two nonagenarian señores vacationing in the forest, one previously Peru's discus representative in the 1948 Olympics in London and the other formerly the country's armed forces' sprint champion. Now, with the old-world courtesy of a forgotten era, the brothers Consigliere tell me as I take their autographs that they are on their way to a new record, being the proud holders of five double by-pass operations between them.

'See what happens with too much exercise?' comments La Señora darkly when later I tell her the tale.

I move on to Tarapoto to sample *la selva alta*, the high rainforest. Again the tranquillity, the detachment from reality. On the hill above the village of Chanca, where the reed-roofed, blankwalled houses are without windows to preclude the ingress of evil spirits, small boys fly their kites in the late-evening breeze. Sky-borne symbols of detachment, free spirits tugging at the umbilical cord. It is the dry season and on the homeward way we cross a dormant watercourse of arid boulders and shingle.

'Here is *el río* Cumbaza,' guide Edgardo informs me, indicating the empty river bed. 'But in this moment without the water. For it is now the dry season and the land he is very droughtie.'

I am reminded of the waterless water feature in the Clinic and of the need to end our own drought.

In the remoteness of my rainforest refuge a radio message is received saying my planned return flight has been cancelled. No real reason, just a passing lack of interest somewhere along the trail. It is *la manera selvática*, the way of the forest. I am advised that I must curtail my visit to take an earlier plane. For once I have a better idea and do nothing, swinging gently in the *hamaca*, the thoughtfully provided hammock on the balcony of my *choza*, my isolated bungalow, watching the ever-changing sky and breathing the whisper of the treetops in the wind. Perhaps there will be a flight tomorrow, or maybe the day after. I suspect I may have imbibed *chamico*, that supernatural potion of the forest of unknown ingredients whose mystical powers will entrap me here until the end of my days and beyond, until the moon is no more.

Certainly as I pass back through Tarapoto I replenish my stocks of *uña de gato*, as recommended by Dr Hermogenes, in case of any forthcoming aches and pains, and whilst inside the dimly lit shop the shaman or *curandero*, the magical medicine man, invites me to invest in a phial of persuasive *pusanga*, and wishes me good fortune with that seductively soft smile of *la selva*. 'Oh, and by the way, did you ever fly with *ayahuasca*, the rope of death?' enquires the mystical medicine man. But I am content to leave some of the secrets of *la selva* intact.

By chance, my eventual appearance back at the Clinic coincides with the hour and the bird from the cuckoo clock hanging in Reception emerges disconcertingly to chide my tardy return. I make to apologize for being several days behind schedule, but happily La Señora, doyenne of *la hora peruana*, is in sympathy with the situation.

'Don't worry,' she says consolingly, 'this clock it is five minutes fast. Anyway, where have you been?'

'Not a boa in sight, not an anaconda to be seen,' I tell her. 'Apart from the snake dancing with the *Booraa*, that is.'

207

She looks at me suspiciously and then gives me that greeting reserved for all vacationers on their reluctant return to the office.

'Well, we have been working busy whilst you have been busy enjoying. During the time you were in the jungles, to the Bank I have been talking with the General Manager of Risk.'

What an excellent title.

'Yes, I went to the Bank, but I was foreign. They were not sure of me. I said to this General Manager of Risk, "You don't remember me, because the day before that I came to see you, you were not there".'

'Quite.'

'Now he says that we need to tie up our pants.'

'What?'

'Tighten the belt. Do less travelling. I laugh at him, but of course, just from within the inside. However, I think there is something wrong there in the opinion. Poor man, he is called Girdleball. Señor Girdleball. His family are not with Peruvian beginnings, I believe it may be an English name. When you say, "Good day to you, Señor Girdleball", he looks down. He is ashamed. Maybe he is a secret agent for another government.'

'Definitely.'

'Now I shall tell you about the elections. There is general unease. They are saying they will take four days to count the votes, at first they said four hours. They say four days will give them more time.'

'More time for what?'

'Exactly. The official observers are saying "*No hay clima pre-electoral genuinamente democrático.*" The situation is short of democracy. Anyway, you must meet Señor Girdleball.'

Our new acquaintance, the General Manager of Risk, is pleased to present us with a new finance plan, a tidy twenty per cent per annum over ten years.

'This is very expensive money,' frowns La Señora. 'No

wonder that man was not directing his eyes to me. These bank people have nothing to tie up their lives to. If I die because of this my monument will be my Clinic. Where will their monument be? I cannot explain it exactly but at times I feel we must learn that in life all of us are not made by the same *patrón*. And by the way, the banks have asked that I do not bring you to the meetings any more, they say that you do not understand the system here.'

'You mean they don't like me saying they are robbing us?'

'Yes. It is a compliment, you made them feel uneasy. Now you will be spared the pollution. And the contamination.'

So many hurdles in our lives. It is around this time that we become aware of the syndrome of the disappearing Peruvian, close cousin of the non-happening Peruvian promise. The scenario runs like this:

'We must visit my house in the mountains,' says the disappearing Peruvian grandly (before he disappears). 'We may swim in the pool, take the sun, ride in the hills and even enjoy the local dishes. I mean to say the typical plates of the region, you understand.'

'How awfully kind. I should love to.'

'This weekend? Why not?'

'Perfect. Couldn't be better.'

'We'll do it.'

And you never hear another thing. Not a squeak.

Or perhaps you receive an exploratory professional visit from a neighbouring clinic. There are clear advantages in working conjointly. A pooling of resources, a beneficial extension of services and an increased range of facilities and expertise. Time is spent, lunch is enjoyed.

'Definitely we must affiliate,' says the about-to-disappear Peruvian. 'Our services are complementary, it will be enormously to our mutual benefit. And to the patients'.'

'Enormously. Marvellous. Let's do it.'

You never hear another thing. Nothing happens.

Or yet another banker will arrive with proposals for yet another financial package. Long meetings, all the figures, all the papers on the table.

'That's fine then,' says the new man from the new bank. 'By tomorrow at the very latest you shall have details of the deal, a longer term, lower rates, a softer loan, a better life.'

Then he disappears, swallowed up by the same black hole that has devoured countless others. We are left to wonder, how can this be?

Just three examples? No, hundreds, enough to fill a book. A monotonous book.

The stage is set for the election, every building, every wall plastered with posters.

'I shall put the music,' says La Señora, turning on the car radio. 'That way I do not have to read the announces.'

On the eve of polling all bars are closed, the sale of liquor prohibited. Shrewd, worthy of emulation. Except that in the best restaurants, beer and wine continue to find their way to favoured clients, poured from innocuous flowery teapots and sipped from equally disarming floral teacups. The international electoral observers say that no, things haven't got any better and that's disappointing, but yes, the elections can go ahead. Difficult to stop them, that's the point. Voting is compulsory, those who fail to perform their civic duty will be fined. Countdown, the final rallies are held, more resembling folk music festivals than fervent political gatherings. It is not the Peruvian way to be too serious for long; everyone is happier with a touch of singing and dancing, including the candidates.

The great day dawns. The field is unchanged: a flock of no-hopers behind the two main contenders. El Chino, the Japanese-by-birth President and unconstitutional candidate for an illegal third term of office, and El Cholo, the challenging indigenous economist. The 14 million voters come and go and at four o'clock sharp the booths close. The results of three independent exit polls are flashed to the nation. All are agreed: about 48 per cent for El Cholo, around 43 per cent for El Chino. Shock result, notwithstanding the chicanery, the people have opted for change. One hour later, more chicanery, more change. The forecasts are reversed, El Chino leads El Cholo. Curious. An earnest announcer explains how these things can happen.

Then it is learnt that by strange misfortune some of the ballot papers had totally omitted El Cholo from the list of candidates. 'Just an unfortunate printing error,' comes the explanation. 'It smells bad,' says *El Comercio*, the honest voice of reason, 'very bad.' El Cholo feels the same. He thinks it smells rotten. Donning a Rambo-style headband he leads thousands of supporters to protest in the city centre. The international observers froth that they are not happy with what they see, the protests continue for three days and El Chino's figures inch inexorably if inexplicably to the requisite 51.5 per cent for a first-round victory. The villain of the piece is the capricious electoral computer. This special computer, put it to bed at night when you are tired of counting votes for the day and wake up in the morning to a different answer, always in favour of El Chino. The cutting edge of technology.

Finally the Government gets the message from the international community. To avoid putting vital aid programmes into jeopardy and the possibility of other economic difficulties, it is accepted it would be a good idea to stage *una segunda vuelta*, a re-match between the two leading players. The tension eases and for another seven weeks the country must revert to electoral campaigning, all over again. More intense now, less colour, less fun, no invisible Ezequiel, no gay horses.

'Don't be downhearted,' says La Señora. 'I have good news for you.' I wait, without expectation. 'You will have no more fourth-floor visitors disturbing your work.' I do nothing to encourage the conversation. 'I have told everyone that you have tendencies.'

'You mean . . . '

'Yes. Anyway, after your Carnival performance, everyone knew.'

'Alicia Alonso was your idea.'

'I can't remember. Also, I have told everyone you have gone bankrupt. And that you have left a trail of abandoned wives and orphans across the seven continents of the world.'

'That should do the trick nicely.'

'Hopefully so, but if necessary, I can easily be even more imaginative. We will explain that you are a resident patient here, undergoing long-term medication and addiction therapy. My other good news is that we are going quickly to Arequipa. There is a family funding possibility that has arisen for the Clinic. I am not available for further questioning, but yes, this may change our lives. We must wait and see. Now you may look up the Colca Canyon in your book.'

'The famed Colca Canyon,' says the guide book, 'Valley of Wonders and home to the giant Andean condor. Reached through the town of Chivay, four hours' drive north of Arequipa.' At an altitude nearing 12,000 feet the height is not an inducement for La Señora.

'My heart it doesn't want to go too high, it beats too much,' she complains.

But go we do, the possibility of rearranging the Clinic loan is paramount. In the 'white city', La Señora undertakes her familial consultations, then, the overtures completed, we take to the road, stopping on the journey to drink the favoured *maté de coca* to combat *soroche*, altitude sickness.

'We do not have to be afraid of the *coca*,' advises La Señora. 'This is a country built on *coca*. In fact I feel very great with the tea. I have discovered that this tea is excellent.'

In the distance are clusters of the vulnerable vicuña, their melancholy eyes reflecting the sadness of the princess trapped within their beings from the days of time indefinite until the end of time. That's according to the legend, and undoubtedly the sad princess was also young and beautiful. Nearer to hand and less nervous are grazing groups of guilt-ridden llamas, undisturbed by their unromantic place in history. Whether the coarse conquistador gave the scrofulous syphilis to the unsuspecting llama who in turn gave it to the innocent Indian, or whether the depraved Indian was the cause of the llama infecting the deprived conquistador depends on who is telling the story. However, history definitely inclines in favour of the Indian and is unequivocal about the central role of the unfortunate llama. The undefiled alpaca with their much-sought-after wool ('Once you get enrolled in the alpaca mood you can't get out of it') complete the trinity.

Arriving at our destination we follow the guide book, admiring the colourful traditional clothing of the ladies of Chivay ('In this group the women all wear long skirts for modesty; of course, what happens under the skirts nobody knows'), visiting the historic churches of the region, absorbing the staggering natural beauty of the canyon with its mosaic of terraced fields, bathing in the hot springs of the Colca Lodge (undeterred and untroubled by the cold rain). Finally we catch our breath and are deprived of speech by the soaring grace and awesome magnificence of the fantastic flight of the huge condors.

'The Incas they were here in the year 1450,' explains La Señora. 'When you in your country were fighting, we were drinking *maté de coca* and waiting for the condor to pass.' Seized by the moment, La Señora is further inspired. 'The success of our Clinic shall be as the effortless flight of the condors,' she exclaims, 'ever upwards. Now we also must fly and go at once to Lima to fulfil our destiny. And by the way, I think I may be successful soon in rearranging our loan. It will be a family matter, no paperwork.'

'¡*Mamasita linda!* Gordon Bennett! That's fantastic! Fantastic! Can you say more?'

'What?' La Señora's attention has been diverted by the ringing of one of her cellulars.

So, wing our way to Lima we do, with condor-like determination. Although first we are detained in Arequipa for a day by an unexpected diversion.

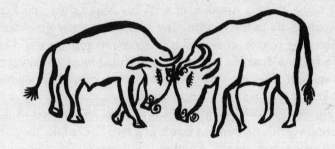

17

Grandes y Tradicionales Peleas de Toros

By chance and good fortune our return from the Colca Canyon takes us through Arequipa on the very day of 'The Grand and Traditional Fights of the Bulls', an annual event, pre-dating *los conquistadores*. 'Unique not only in Peru, not only in South America, but in the entire world', with origins in the timeless local manner of settling rural disputes: your bull against my bull. It is supposedly peculiar to Arequipa because of the 'exceptional aridity of the climate mixed with an abundance of solar radiation which induces terrible negative feelings in the bulls'. Try to move the event to Lima or export it to Argentina and it's a flop. Nothing happens. A total insufficiency of terrible negative feelings. Except, interestingly, for the remoteness of northern Bangladesh, where pre-monsoon climatic conditions invoke the same symptoms and the sport flourishes. Uniqueness is a rare and fragile flower.

It is the event's Announcer with his heavy-duty speakers who alerts us to the contest. The lady gatekeeper gives us a welcoming nod, a smile and a programme and we stand on the edge of a dusty field fringed with the ubiquitous eucalyptus and a milling crowd of at least a dozen other aficionados. It is *la hora peruana*. The Announcer sends a messenger over to obtain my personal details which in turn are relayed to the waiting world. As things are running two hours late, they are short of fresh material. Anything will serve. The throng of spectators, now swollen to fifty, eye me with curiosity on hearing the untruth that I have come all the way from London to attend. This is veritably an International Event affirms the Announcer, not letting the facts stand in the way of a good story.

From the Grandstand, an elevated platform accommodating twenty empty plastic chairs for officials, wives, mistresses and other dignitaries, there is a good view of the arena, also empty except for three mounted policemen and a boy with a lime green T-shirt and a yo-yo. As three o'clock nears, the gathering grows to several hundred, with many more pressing through the gate. My neighbour says the hour has come, and things look promising as the field is cleared of stragglers, with the exception of the lime green boy. The Announcer's commentary approaches fever pitch.

I buy a ticket for the *Gran Rifa*. First prize in the raffle is tethered to the front of the Grandstand. One black-faced sheep, live, beribboned. Second prize (not on view): A sack of rice; third prize: Noodles. There is a rustic purity about this raffle.

An expectant hush heralds the opening contest. Master and Macanazo are the two adversarial bulls, weighing in at 600 kilograms but in comparison to later contestants just the featherweights of the afternoon's entertainment. They are cajoled and tickled into position by their handlers, much pawing and bellowing prefacing the ultra-fierce contest to come. But it is not to be. Master stands stolidly centre-field, ready to be half-interested if the situation warrants, Macanazo keeps his distance, circling sulkily and avoiding eye contact. The tight-jeaned crowd are silent in disbelief, the handlers tickle to no avail. Suddenly, Macanazo trots briskly through the exit. It is decisive. Not a shot fired and it's all over. Master is led triumphant from the field, smirking arrogantly.

'The next one will be better,' says my neighbour, in case I too am about to head for the exit. Nube Negra and Alma Negra, Black Cloud and Black Soul, take to the field purposefully, balls swinging jauntily, set to restore the good name of the illustrious occasion after the last debacle. More rising dust, the handlers and the friends and associates of the handlers retire to a respectful distance, whilst the protagonists lock horns, shove, heave and shove again. The bevy of judges, earnest men in white, appraise the performance critically, at times on bended knee to detect finer points of detail and subtleties of technique.

After ten minutes of grappling I find myself scanning the programme and counting the number of battles still to come, wondering if Nube or Alma might oblige with a heart attack. Everyone else, right down to the last pair of pointed boots, is riveted to the occasion. Then, summoned by some unseen bell or gong, pitched beyond the reach of human hearing, Cloud and Soul give each other one final contemptuous eyeballing and canter from the field of play, as though in need of refreshing tea and toast. The judges confer, the spectators head back to the beer tent. The well-packed jeans promenade to and fro contentedly in front of the Grandstand. The final verdict goes to Cloud. Or was it Soul? Nobody seems too concerned.

However, when we reach *El Estelar*, the Big Fight of the day, or rather, evening, the mood has changed. The lime green boy with the yo-yo has long gone home and sun is setting. In all Arequipa and its environs, overlooked by Chachani, Pichu

Pichu and Misti, the three majestic volcanoes, only in this grassless little field is the temperature rising. This is the time of the heavyweights, tipping the scales at a nonchalant 1,300 kilograms apiece. We are not to be disappointed. Camerún and Apagón strain like constipated leviathans, a battle royal. Up goes the dust, down go the heads, horns implacably locked. The judges are all on one knee now, heedless of the laundry bill. This one is going to be difficult. But slowly, slowly, Camerún seems to be getting the upper hand, or horn. Yes, imperceptible at first, but Camerún is undeniably ahead on points. Suddenly, sensation. Apagón flips Camerún on his back, the throw of the afternoon, and takes full advantage of the situation; always kick a man when he is down. Camerún's eyes water and we wince in sympathy. Apagón turns to the judges. You decide, he tells them. Camerún concurs. The judges look uncomfortable. They eye the handlers and supporters uncertainly. Bets have been placed, money is at stake. The Announcer tries a few bars of inappropriate music and the three mounted policemen move centre stage in hope of some light entertainment. The judges deliberate, heads bowed. They try and edge unobtrusively towards the exit, wishing themselves invisible but observed by two thousand pairs of eyes. The music stops. The Announcer gives the verdict.

'A draw!' he declares.

A draw! After all that, 2,600 heaving kilograms of it, and they say it's a draw?

'Yes, it's a draw,' says my neighbour equably. He motions to the bulls. 'They drew,' he explains.

So, the money stays where it is or goes back to where it started, except for a handful of smart nuevos soles correctly wagered on the unlikely and inconclusive outcome. The mounted policemen withdraw, disappointed. No fighting. The black-faced raffle prize looks on impassively. The perfect end to a perfect day. The judges toss a coin, the heads bow again as it falls to the ground. The destiny of that magnificent trophy determined by the spin of a coin. Everybody is happy, that's the way it is. Worse than a penalty shoot-out. New perspectives.

The lady gatekeeper gives us a nod, a farewell smile and another programme, just in case. She has a few spare. That night I lie awake and wait for the knock on the door. Will it be the black-faced sheep, the fat sack of rice or the box of noodles? But the midnight knock never comes. Our priority now is to hurry back to Lima to resuscitate the ailing Clinic, taking heart from the muscular endeavour of the monolithic bulls as well as the soaring condors. And possibly absorbing a handful of those terrible negative feelings, all the better to do battle with the Bank.

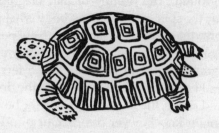

18

Voy y Vengo – I Go and I Come

The days have slipped past. Inexorably the weeks have turned into months. And the months? Who knows how many have drifted by, like ethereal clouds passing over the dead tree in the garden? The idyll of my entanglement with The Ladies' Healthcare Clinic, Lima has assumed a timeless quality. But idyll or not, it is time to visit England. In the modern world, travel as far as you like, life's administrative irritations are sure to follow. In any case, it is mid-April and my imagined mountain of Christmas cards has too long been gathering dust on the London doormat. As for Peru, soaring condors and heaving monolithic bulls aside, it is a good moment for distance to work its enchanting spell, to put a new perspective on my astigmatic friends, the prurient pigeons. Especially now that the cloudy clag of mildewed winter is fast descending over Lima, enveloping flowery Miraflores.

'Don't worry,' says La Señora, 'I will come to Inglaterra with you.'

How did she know I was worrying? I wasn't but I am now. I discover an unexpected ally. The bank manager advises firmly against such a plan. La Señora is crestfallen; I find myself looking at the grey man in a different light.

'Take care of everything while I am gone,' I exhort. 'And don't forget to finalize the Arequipa loan! Then we can get the lift, finish the waterfall, and open the clinics for the poor. And you can start painting again!'

Arriving in Battersea, I am accorded the traditional warm-hearted British welcome. At the entrance to my flat, ancient Ivy, the unromantically styled cleaner of common parts, twines herself around her mop and eyes me doubtfully.

'Oh, we're back, are we?' she observes accusingly, with a marked lack of enthusiasm.

'Back we are,' I confirm apologetically, heaving an appropriately heavy sigh, *in flagrante delicto* and unable to deny the obvious. Once inside with the kettle on I ring my friends.

'What?' they ask. 'Pru who?' Then they tell me that the weather has been quite dreadful recently. Occasionally the response is more animated. 'We thought you were dead,' says one sepulchral soul.

All is not lost and I settle easily to springtime London. Apart from the telephone calls. La Señora is master, or mistress, of the plaintive message. Pathos, that's her speciality. No one could fail to be moved by the tragic tale of my empty office. In my absence, the sad Señora advises, the Clinic is suffering from an acute case of 'failure to thrive', and unless I return immediately, things will be dire indeed. But I detect an acute case of hyperbole and stand firm. That's until the launch of the campaign of calling in the small hours of the morning, for me, truly the dead of night. Global time zones are a bothersome detail of no concern to La Señora. She rings from her office at eight in the evening, the last of the Doctor's patients homeward bound, unwilling to acknowledge that it is two in the morning for the law-abiding citizens of Inglaterra. I fumble for the telephone, ready to capitulate. Can the early-morning knock on the door be far behind?

'You sound strange,' comments my Peruvian pursuer.

'No, fine, thank you,' I lie. 'Positively dandy.'

'Are you busy in this moment?' she enquires. 'Are you alone?'

'No, not busy,' I answer, truthfully.

'Then I will give you the news.' And she does. About those unspeakable people in the Bank, always pressing, life in the Clinic with the fourth floor abandoned, empty, even derelict. But Dr Desastre is well. Very well, actually. More popular than ever. I resist the temptation to enquire after his diet sheets for the horses. But Clinic costs are rising, revenue is static. Plus ça change. No further word on the family loan. That's depressing. And oh yes, Lupi Pancho, the deranged electrician, has confusingly cross-connected the front door entry-phone with the Clinic fax machine. Everything is normal. 'I need your character urgent,' she concludes. 'Come quickly.'

Perhaps I might just send my character and remain, characterless, in London. After several harassing nights, La Señora plays her ace.

'Be careful,' I am told. 'Lose your place for too long and you may come back and find your bed busy.'

'What about the church choir here?' I ask. 'They need me.'

'You can sing in Peru,' says La Señora down the midnight phone. 'I sang in my school. I was the second voice. I was very good on that. Like a cannery.'

Canaries are persuasive birds. Jorge Chávez beckons.

I land in Lima and from the remoteness of the unproductive baggage carousel scan the waiting throng of relatives and well-wishers gathered without. I wave in hope. Everybody waves back. But for me, there is no one. There is no sign of La Señora or the Doctor. Equally, there is no sign of my suitcase.

'Maybe your bag might arrive tomorrow,' declares the airline person, reluctantly and reaching for the *subjuntivo*. 'It happens sometimes.' Clearly not if they can help it.

'*Hasta mañana*,' I say to the guard, resignedly, and go outside to find a taxi.

'*Sí*,' he replies. 'Until tomorrow.' Déjà vu déjà vu, obviously.

The taxi bargaining commences. Twenty dollars? No. Ten dollars? *No, gracias*. Fifteen nuevos soles? That's more like it, a quarter of the first offer. But the driver hasn't given up yet. Right, he says, so that will be twenty nuevos soles with the tax. What tax is that? Welcome back to Lima, Peru.

Off we set through the traffic, all those erratic combi mini-buses, about 13,000 of them, all those pollution-belching trucks, number unknown. This year there is no El Niño to disturb the weather patterns and the June blanket of winter cloud hangs heavy over the city. Lima the Grey, the curse of the Incas. It is Christmas weather, a time for candles and log fires. The scarlet poinsettias are in full bloom. Perhaps the countries of the southern hemisphere should seek ecclesiastical dispensation to celebrate the Nativity six months out of phase.

We arrive at the Clinic. The taxi driver is impressed with the grandeur of my Miraflores home, but is unable to devise a means of relating this to an increase in the fare. A new security guard greets me at the front door, introducing himself as

Cirilon Max Factor Yupanqui, at your service. With a name like that he should be standing for President. For the moment he contents himself with wearing the smartest pair of striped wedding trousers on the block. A touch tight under the armpits, otherwise a most enviable fit.

Cirilon Max Factor Yupanqui informs me that Mighty Manolo, our previous diminutive *vigilante*, has not yet exactly passed on, but has gone home to rest and to prepare for the possibility of such an occurrence. I send my *saludos*. Hopefully they will arrive in time.

'And what about our other guard,' I enquire, 'Alfredo is well?'

'Er, señor, you perhaps mean Alberto?'

'Yes, of course. Alberto! How is Alberto?'

'*Lamentablemente* he is not so well. He is in special care. He is in a home.'

'Really? Why?'

'Well, you always called him Alfredo, and La Señora always called him Alfonso. Then she started calling him Alfresco. Then Dr Hermogenes called him Francesco. And all the time he was Alberto.'

'I see. Tricky, hmmm?'

'*Sí*, señor, tricky for Alfonso. He had an identity crisis followed by a nervous breakdown. Now we have Florentino.'

'Right. What did you say your name was again?'

As I enter the Clinic, Ernestina looks out from under the stairs, readily distracted from the lure of the ledgers. She is wearing headphones, a mouthpiece and a long aerial, like a Martian switchboard operator. In the excitement of seeing me, the aerial gets entangled with the stairs and the headset falls over her eyes. To spare her blushes, I go up to Reception, only to find Nurse Dulce similarly attired. Snap! Martians everywhere! Her eyes fill with the joy of my return, then she remembers her *Star Wars* apparel and vanishes. Moving upwards, ever upwards, I meet Señorita Hilda in the auditorium. Snap again!

'The new intercom system,' she explains tersely, and with a flick of her aerial she beams herself on her way as I nod sympathetically. Up the final flight of stairs and I check my office to ensure my absence has not provoked the syndrome of the disappearing desk. It's still there, a bad omen; it means no one else wanted it. But what's this? Signs of female occupancy. Fragrant clues, tissues instead of dust, flowers on the desk. Ominous.

There have been other innovations during my shorter-than-expected absence. The hand of the International Shopper is much in evidence: several new items of furniture on the landings and decorating the passageways, solicitous sofas like motorway lay-bys, arms akimbo, in case anyone should need temporary respite after the exertion of taking nine or ten consecutive paces, additional curtains, tasselled tie-backs, attractive rugs of Middle Eastern provenance overlying the fitted carpets.

From the vantage point of my bedroom balcony, I spot a large placard in the auditorium proudly announcing 'The John M. Lane Institute of Hospital and Clinic Administration', and there is an accompanying mound of similarly inscribed T-shirts with a passable likeness of bespectacled John M. Lane on the back, bearing a curious resemblance to an astigmatic pigeon. At the moment, my return is evoking more questions than answers. My confused attention is then further diverted as I see through the window that, sadly, most of my potted flowers, palms and shrubs are comprehensively dead, a sorry sight. La Señora had warned me in advance that there had been a slight problem, an overdose of kindness. The impulsively caring Royal Horticultural Society member for Lima has been generous to a fault with the fertilizer.

Providentially, and saving further astonishment, my tour of

inspection is interrupted by the flurrying arrival of La Señora herself, like the theatre curtain rising on gala night.

'Oh!' she exclaims. 'You took a taxi! How awful!'

'No, yes,' I protest, unconvincingly. 'It was a very fine taxi. Four wheels. Not even a Tico. The driver was a former Minister of the Economy.'

'I had flowers for you, but I was closely assaulted at the airport.'

La hora peruana. Be thankful that La Señora got the day right.

'I have made many changes here,' she tells me, unnecessarily. 'Your old Land Rover is repaired but you cannot put him to work too much on account of his age. And the dried-up *catarata* for the relaxing prenatal ladies is now with water, it just needs a new whose.'

'Ah! A hose!'

'Speak Spanish please,' directs La Señora crossly. Then she continues. 'Anyway, it is my personal class and it is a success. Also, thinking forward to the future, we have a new nurse, Dolores, who will work with Nurse Dulce, but she is very shied.'

I bite my tongue and nod comprehendingly. I am not falling into that trap again.

'I thought it best to get another nurse, in case we get the loan and then the lift. Also, we have a new Executive Controller. She is my Aunt Gertrudis actually and she will share your office. In fact, she started work last week, but I have learnt that after her lunch she cannot get up the stairs, so possibly she will not persist. Anyway, here you can see that we have been running all the moment.'

'Yes indeed. Everything is brilliant. Er, I note that we have formed a new Institute . . . '

'Yes. In Peru we can do anything, so I just did that. You may give a Seminar next week. And I have thrown away all your clothes.'

'Brilliant. Sorry? You have done what?'

'Yes, don't suffer for that, you need a new wardrobe, a new image for the Millennium.'

I do now. 'Thank you. I feel you are right.' I think about my missing suitcase. I have always tried to travel light. Another dream come true.

La Señora loses interest in that topic. 'Now we have a party for you. The only thing is we are waiting for the moment to celebrate and to put the music. Come!'

That night I don't sleep as well as I might. There is an earthquake at about four in the morning. Just a tremor, the epicentre some way distant. I wonder if the next devastation of a Lima earthquake will be in my lifetime or will it coincide with the end of it? I am not enamoured of earthquakes, but in truth my mind is on my empty wardrobe. Not even space in the heavens above can rival the void of an unused wardrobe, coldly reproachful, forlorn, abandoned and bored, the jumbled hangers huddled defiant and unclothed at the far end of the rail. A search (yes, frantic) has revealed an overlooked pair of shorts at the back of one drawer, two socks and a beach shirt in another. To that I can add one toothbrush, half a packet of Old English toffees and a good book. Hardly an excess of riches, but there are people with less. A second tremor curtails my thinking. The Clinic sways, my framed photograph (unsigned) of heroic Bert Trautman this time falls from the bedside table, fortunately without breaking, and I survey my humble possessions. Dead plants, empty cupboards, missing baggage: these are the minutiae of life. It is time to move up the Richter scale, to be positive. Fate has tailored my circumstances, and my wardrobe. I can only travel in one direction: to *el gimnasio* at Village Dasso.

227

Walking to Dasso, I see my surroundings with fresh eyes. The amorous doves and the misbehaving parrots are still overhead in the treetops, the abounding flowers of Miraflores are much in evidence in spite of the winter solstice, the high-rise buildings are similarly sprouting but with unwelcome vigour. The same enervated, resentful Indians are lounging at the same street corners.They came from the mountains to find fortune in Lima. No one said anything about work. If you want land, take it. Take anything you need. Fair shares for all. Don't ask why the economy is up the spout, that's all. They stare accusingly as I pass, countenances carrying the shadow of doom. I gaze back with the clear conscience of a man wearing his only pair of socks with half a packet of toffees in his only pair of shorts. Welcome to Lima, Peru, where they plant new lawns by hand, blade by blade. No seeds, three men to do the job: one to watch, one to talk about nothing, and one actually putting the grass into the ground, root by root. An eloquent commentary on the availability of labour and time.

'¡Hola!' comes the greeting from my friends at the gym, those getting in shape to look good on the beach whilst they get a tan to look good in the gym whilst they are preparing for the beach. 'Are you fitted?'

'Well, not so much,' I admit. 'But soon I will be fitted again.'

I am relieved that I seem to have been forgiven for the shameful incident of the sugar-coated doughnuts. Not only that, I had forgotten how good everyone looks in their leotards. Carmencita, Teresita, Fabiolita, Charapita, Tortalita, Lillianita, Cecilita, Rominita, Ingridsita, Sashacita: divine creatures, celestial bodies all. I struggle with my work-out; it is more a matter of concentration than a question of not being fitted. The heavenly firmament apart, I am also preoccupied with more earthly considerations, such as those static patient numbers and the vacant upstairs nursing suites in the Clinic. In due course I head for Casa Bonomini in search of further news and, failing that, replacement calories.

The Fathers' Day breakfast, another overseas importation, is in full flow. All the family are present, La Señora and Dr Hermogenes presiding. Gleaming Margarita, big and black, who nearly broke Papá Noel's leg on Christmas Eve, is happy at the jovial stove. Abraham, the scissor-dancing artilleryman, has donned a waiter's jacket and is tending the laden table.

'What has become of Bruno, the other butler?' I enquire.

'We think he accelerated Fathers' Day and is still in the bed,' states La Señora darkly.

The surviving Yorkshire terriers are excited and underfoot.

'Disgusting little dogs,' growls Medical Student One. 'They should definitely pass to a better life.'

Out on the lawn is Fidel, the non-blooming gardener, watering the tortoise. He and Carlotta share the same expression, communing in static, or ecstatic, silence. Fidel always visits the house on high days and holidays.

'*Hoy día es un día laborable para mi*, today is a working day for me,' he will tell you proudly, to foster the illusion that in the horticultural industry (of which, note well, he is a senior representative) the ever-changing seasons and the thrusting new shoots wait for no man. Then, to emphasize his point, he adds rhetorically with sly innocence: 'And are you not yourself working today?' Actually, he is forever hoping to find the house without the owners in residence, so that he may spend a few memorable moments of prime time hoeing and sowing with shapely Señorita María Milagro, the obligingly succulent maid from *la sierra*.

More immediately, few know that Carlotta the tortoise is in deep disgrace. She has not been invited to the party. It is a fresh skeleton in the family cupboard, leaving a less than fresh odour. It is difficult to say how good is Carlotta's eyesight, but probably not very. Maybe all right to drive a car but not to fly an aeroplane. It so happens that the dogs' supper dish is in the shape of a tortoise shell, and Carlotta was discovered, or rather surprised, late one night by Medical Student One, mounted on the aforesaid dish, breathing heavily. Naturally, we all wish it hadn't happened. La Señora in particular, matriarch and guardian of the noble lineage, has taken it hard. Like dubious defence lawyers, we tell her that it is an isolated lapse, quite out of character, but she is not to be consoled or convinced.

'Maybe Carlotta should be surgeried,' she suggests pensively, with just a hint of menacing retribution. In no time at all the vet is summoned and spends time alone with the disgraced carapace. He emerges from behind closed doors with stern mien to give his diagnosis to the gathered family, anxiously waiting without.

'Hot water?' they enquire. 'More hot water?' The vet nods in affirmation.

'It's a boy,' he pronounces. 'Congratulations.'

'*¡Dios santo!* And *miércoles!* A boy?'

'Yes, she's a he.'

Dios santo indeed! Only a swift inhalation of the smelling salts is sufficient to save the swooning Señora. Of course, I knew it all along, but I hold my tongue. People who say 'I told you so' don't go to heaven. Carlotta the transvestite tortoise! *¡Que escándalo!* The application of science to resolve the mysteries of life, for example to determine the existence or otherwise of pixies, elves and fairies, or the Loch Ness Monster, or to ascertain the gender of a tortoise, is not always for the best. Notwithstanding, for want of a better alternative, the tempo of the Fathers' Day breakfast resumes.

Elderly Aunt Gertrudis, elegance personified and until quite recently the Executive Controller of The Ladies' Healthcare Clinic, Lima, greets me effusively, although like Carlos, the rechristened tortoise, she is also acting out of character. It must be the weather. She is clutching a half-drunk bottle of beer. She looks almost as though she might have been swigging the contents. Except that graceful Aunt Gertrudis never swigged anything in her life.

'Welcome back to Lima, Peru,' she tells me.

'I am happy to be back in Lima, Peru,' I assure her, catching the cadence.

I am brought up to date on the political scene. Now we definitely have a *dictadura*.

'Peru is like a tomato in a hot pot boiling,' explains La Señora graphically. 'One day it will explode and all the seeds will be flattered against the wall.' So many prophecies, so much truth.

The second round of voting was won in familiarly doubtful circumstances by ineligible El Chino. So upset was El Cholo with the continuing chicanery that he tucked the electoral ball under his arm and refused to play, instructing his supporters not to vote. He has been protesting ever since, but, says La Señora, he may have tripped himself up with his own bootlaces. He dreams of a third round of voting but it seems a forlorn hope. Or is it?

'El Cholo knew he was lost,' say the pundits, 'and El Chino wants to be a maximum hero. Why, we can't tell. Although maybe one day we will learn the dark secrets. It is not necessary for him to persist. Already to open and close the doors of his car he has enough people.'

The long-suffering, weary electorate appear to have accepted the status quo. They have lives to lead, there is football to be watched, fiestas to attend. There will be another election in five years' time, so what's all the fuss about?

The minor matter of the one million false votes? The investigation has been completed. It transpires it was all the work of a few misguided junior clerks acting on their own misaligned initiative without, thankfully, any involvement of higher officials. No prosecutions or further action will be necessary. Of course not. I learn that various international bodies are scheduled to arrive to deliver their verdict on events in Peru, and that El Cholo has promised a massive protest to coincide with El Chino's official re-reinstallation in office. Hopefully involving nothing more than a few broken windows and a few bruised heads.

'We are a people of passivity,' I am advised. 'A little movement here and there, then we carry on.'

It is enough of politics. Except to hear that by way of protest, La Señora went to the polls dressed in fuchsia shoes, baggy black pantaloons, a clown's green and yellow smock, a violent violet fuzzy wig and a big red nose with '*Esto es un Circo*' emblazoned on her back. 'This is a Circus': it was what nobody else was brave enough to say. Not content with that, La Señora also found room on her commodious T-shirt to write 'NO to Fraud' and 'We need a Peruvian President who can speak Castellano'. Then comes the sad news: the non-campaigning presidential candidate, invisible Ezequiel, has died. His protest was the most emphatic of all.

'I am not so concerned with politics,' declares one not-so-certain voice from the far end of the late-breakfast gathering.

The answer comes swift and sure. 'It is your country, it is all around you. You have no choice, you are involved. It is happening. Here you cannot choose which pieces of life to select, like cakes on a plate.'

'Democracy in Peru is a corpse,' writes a recently departed ambassador, delivering his verdict with the authority of high office and the candour of distance and retirement. But it is La Señora who has the final say.

'All this,' she tells us dismissively, 'is but a minor paragraph in the history of Peru.'

A little later La Señora appears at my elbow to divulge a further item of news.

'Tomorrow we shall go to Ecuador,' she reveals. 'We must be

at the airport at four in the morning. I am teaching you the surprise life. Prepare your luggage. Clean shoes and socks with no holes. Now I have to run some errands.'

'But, but . . . what about the Seminar?'

But she has gone. Anyway, I haven't got any socks, with or without holes. And why should we visit Ecuador? The only thing for it is to go and find out. At least packing won't be a problem.

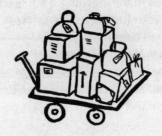

19

Vamos y Venimos – We Go and We Come

The flight to Quito is at dawn. One day we will find an aeroplane that leaves after a good breakfast. But not this one. The pilot is keen to be on his way.

'Do we really want to be at the airport at four a.m.? That's crazy!'

'It is an obligation by the Government,' replies La Señora flatly.

If I could have commanded obedience from the relevant muscles I would have raised an eyebrow. Instead, I gamble and order a taxi to be at the Clinic at five. In the event, it arrives on time and it is raining. Not yet sunrise and already two surprises.

'How many are you?' enquires the *taxista*.

'I am one,' I reply helpfully. 'But one more is to come.'

The driver nods in puzzlement, defeated by the mathematics. Ex-Ministers of the Economy abound. We drive the short distance to Casa Bonomini. No surprises here. The house is in pitch darkness as though in readiness for an air raid. I ring. And ring. Finally sleepy Señorita Silvia appears from the gloom, the maid of the week. Sometimes we have a maid for a day, sometimes for a month. It depends on how long they choose to stay before filling a plastic bag with all that they can carry and fleeing.

Eventually an enormous suitcase emerges into the half light propelled by La Señora, dwarfed by her belongings. Lucky for some, for instance those whose baggage hasn't been misplaced on a previous journey and whose remaining possessions haven't been consigned to the trash can. After all, we will be in Ecuador for almost two entire days. Who knows what invitations to balls and banquets may come our way? I note that La Señora has opted to travel in one of the minks. I hadn't realized that Quito was going to be so cold. I need to check the atlas again. Maybe they made a mistake with the equator. Maybe we are going to another ice sculpture competition.

'You never know how things are,' explains La Señora, reading my thoughts. 'We could land anywhere. When you woke me with the doorbell I said to myself first I will stand up and take a shower, then I will put my clothes on me when I find out where they are. I asked myself what shall I wear today? And somehow I felt for a mink this morning. Never would I wish for anyone to tell me that I am ugly dressed. By the way, are we late?'

'Well . . . ' I begin, thinking of our obligation to the Government. But the question was purely rhetorical.

'Last night there was a dinner. It finished this morning.'

'This morning? We should have travelled tomorrow.'

'Tomorrow? Tomorrow why? But it is true, I am desperate tired.'

Then she falls asleep. If I am patient then I may learn why we are going to Ecuador. But not yet. For the moment it is sufficient to travel hopefully.

La Señora wakes with a start. 'I just remembered. The Doctor told me not to spend any of my money on this trip. None at all.'

Sounds like an excellent prescription to me. The bank manager would have said the same, except he wasn't consulted. But just a moment . . . if La Señora isn't spending any of her money on this trip, whose money will she be using?

'I feel resented,' sighs my companion sadly, and goes back to sleep. I continue to travel hopefully. It is the things you fail to do in this life that you regret more than the things you do. After all, who am I to wonder why I have forsaken the cocooning comfort of my bed to fly to Ecuador?

We are ready to land. Second highest capital in the world, Quito is 9,000 feet above sea level. Not far to drop.

'Thank you for flying us,' announces the stewardess. Thank you too, even the pilot.

There are some two million people in Quito; the airport has an up-country feel. In the car park we have a choice between Taxi Amigo and Taxi Trans Rabbit. We are saved the difficult decision by the arrival of Wilson.

'I am Wilson Sánchez,' says Wilson, formally introducing himself. '*Chofer* and general assistant, I come from Señor Gayo.'

'And now he is giving us the information who is he,' intervenes La Señora helpfully.

'From Miguel Gayo? The famous Spanish painter?'

'*Sí*,' says La Señora. 'He is my *profesor*. If we get the new loan and I have time to paint again, then I must revise my knowledge and handling of the brushes.'

'Goodness gracious! Your teacher! And so famous!'

'Almost. His only problem is that he isn't dead and that the "a" came before the "o". But we don't think on that. We want to lead the life with him. Wilmer will drive us to his atelier now.'

Wilson does. At each set of traffic lights the car is besieged by outstretched hands. It is impossible to gratify them all. We could still be in Lima.

'When God grants you, you need to know how to share,' La Señora reminds us. 'Normally beggars are shied, it is hard to receive as a humble. But these people they beg without shy. You give the hand, they take the elbow.'

If we want, we can buy a pair of reading glasses while the lights are changing, to save visiting the optician. Sweets, choc-olates, magazines, mobile telephones, everything. Quicker than internet shopping, instant delivery through the window, no extra charge.

'That's amazing,' say I.

'What?'

'That people do that.'

'What?'

'Buy their glasses at the traffic lights.'

La Señora adjusts the spectacles on the end of her delicate but noble nose.

'I do,' she says coldly. 'But to be honest,' she admits, 'I find that I am not looking too well. Each day I see less and less.'

I am not surprised. But I have learnt my lesson. Life is for lis-tening.

'These ophthalmologists, the more they put on you, the less you see,' continues La Señora. 'You cannot see, I cannot see; two blinds.'

No, I will not be drawn.

We arrive at the Miguel Gayo studio of art. The great man, bearded and brooding, greets us with gracious warmth, silver-topped cane and flowing cape. We are surrounded by treasure and works of art, not least a Zuloaga and a Toulouse-Lautrec.

It is mid-morning. Brandy is served. Artists do that kind of thing. The conversation flows, olives and cashew nuts are nibbled. And all the time that Frenchman's painting is hanging on the wall. It is like sharing a sacrilegious pizza in a room with Oscar Wilde or Somerset Maugham looking on. Meanwhile, La Señora is seized by the creative atmosphere and sets to work at a handy easel where four handsomely prancing horses soon take shape. Wilson bobs in and out generously with the brandy and dark-eyed ladies with names like Candelaria, Marisol, Paola, Herminia and Anya-Zuleika glide through the salon in tight sweaters to confer and exchange confidences with the maestro.

La Señora lays down her palette. I put down my brandy.

'With Miguel as my professor I take up inspiration like a sponge. But now I am resting away from my paint. It produce me boring. And the latitude.'

'The altitude?'

'That too.' Pause. 'I will make a present of the horses to Winston.'

'I am sure Wilson will be delighted.'

'Now you must choose to buy one or two of Miguel's paints.'

'Paintings? Yes. Why not?' Wilson is at my elbow again with the decanter.

Over the years the Gayo style has had many manifestations. Now he is devoutly abstract, much favoured by the cognoscenti of London, Madrid and New York. La Señora assists me in making my choice.

'To look at these, small your eyes very much and you will see what you see.'

I do and I do. It is difficult to decide which one is best for me, so I take two. La Señora is disappointed. 'Oh, you are not taking the blue,' she sighs. 'The colour of your eyes. This I like a lot.'

'Oh, all right. I'll take the blue. It's nice.'

'English is a language of understatement,' admonishes La Señora. 'Here, "nice" is not enough. You must say more. Find all the superlatives in your head and then you can be on top of the world. And by the way, you cannot leave the red. And of course, this one here you must take.'

So I take three of the Gayo paints. Or is it five? I am happy to share the fame. And to sip the brandy.

Fortuitously, we have arrived in colonial Quito of the conquistadors in the dry season. As the day progresses and we move on to other things, clouds hang heavy on the mountains and unseasonal rain sets in relentlessly. But it's not that cold and throughout our visit I see only one mink coat in the city. La Señora is working to a plan, there is no time for tourism.

'Here in Ecuador,' she declares, 'inflation is one hundred per cent. In four days your breakfast will be one per cent cheaper. Or maybe dearer. Anyway, this is very cheap money and now you are understanding better why we are here. I always benefit from the moment. I am not a shopping person, I am a sort of advantage-mileage person. Here, Watson, stop here please!'

Wilson does as he is bid and pulls up alongside a shop specializing in headstones. I look at La Señora suspiciously. It is one of her recurrent themes.

'Do you have insurance?' she asks repeatedly, sometimes in the middle of lunch, sometimes passing me a note during meetings with the Bank (before the ban). I can see her point: the cost of putting someone in a box and sending them all the way back to London must be on the steep side. We gaze in thoughtful silence through the rain at the shining headstones. I can't help thinking that one of those blocks of stone is going to be mighty heavy to carry to the airport check-in counter. Could be terminal.

However, it seems I have drawn the wrong conclusion. The shop also specializes in handsome brass plaques, ideal for the front door of the Clinic, à la Harley Street. All at a fraction of the Lima price. Inflation definitely has its advantages.

'You see how I benefit from the moment? This will be another very cheap bargain.'

Lighter than a headstone too. La Señora has set the mood for the day. We are investors.

'Here everything is not so expensive. By spending, I am saving.'

'Yes, but . . . ' I should like to meet the author of that slogan.

'What shall we write on the plaque?'

I deliberate. 'How about "The Ladies' Healthcare Clinic, Lima"?'

Now our objective switches to furniture. I watch the mounting mound of chosen merchandise with equally mounting dismay. The advantage-mileage person senses my concern.

'This is not for me,' she explains, 'this is for my house, and for the Clinic, of course. It is good that I do this here, rather than Dr Hermogenes. For the buying of antiques I have the better eye. It is good to invest the new loan even before we get it. That way it will be secure, *sí o no*?'

'But . . . '

'This davenport will serve nicely in case one of the patients should wish to write a letter from the Clinic. Perhaps if the Doctor is delayed. Leonardo will repair the drawer and the varnish and it can go by the window in Reception. Soon we may choose a silver inkstand for company. And this occasional table, mahogany, I think, will support a computer for the waiting husbands, so they can confirm their fortunes on the internet or play simple games with themselves. Chairs are always useful for resting, so we will take those, and these eight Corinthian columns will serve as pedestals for when we buy some more statues. Or we could put busts of famous people on them for the library or somewhere.'

Following distractedly in the slipstream of the great investor, dismissing heretical visions of a row of bullfighters' busts in the auditorium, I wonder whether to buy one of the locally made straw hats from a passing salesman who is pleased to put a succession on my head. Judging by the price, these must surely be the coveted uncrushable reed hats from Montecristi in the province of Manabi mentioned in the guide book. But La Señora is critical.

'You look like a mushroom,' she says, always entertained by her mordant wit.

'A fungus?'

'*Sí*, maybe a toadstool. With glasses.'

Secretly I imagine that I look like Humphrey Bogart, so I complete the purchase.

By chance, we pass the British Embassy.

'I must ring the British Ambassador. I will tell him that I am related to England because of this and that and invite him to meet our group,' says La Señora. 'And I can mention the Clinic. New patients are welcome.'

I am pondering on this in silence when suddenly the embryonic diplomatic hostess exclaims loudly and without warning. 'Elmer! Sorry, Wilmer! Stop the car! Here I am just going to drop my pants.'

'*¿Perdón?*'

'These in this bag for re-mending and organizing.'

For letting out, I suspect. Wilson draws up outside the seamstress's shop.

'I am not letting these pants out,' says La Señora with unsettling intuition. 'I am letting them down. They are too high. I call them my "crossing the river pants". And by the way,' she adds, 'I do so like the way you fit in your hat. You look like Humphrey Bogart.'

As we do the rounds of Quito, La Señora's attention is caught by a succession of graffiti. *'Ecuador – Pobre Tren de Sueños Vendidos'*. The untranslatable phrase keeps popping up. 'Ecuador – Poor Train of Dreams Sold'. Or maybe 'stolen dreams'? 'Poor Ecuador', says another scrawl, 'A Train without Hope'. And again: 'The Bank is Laughing and the People are Dying'. We are in sympathy with that. But La Señora has fixated on the train. She senses an *América Latina* scandal, another case of a disappearing train, just like the proposed commuter train in Lima that never was because someone supposedly eloped with the funds. I suggest that the sentiments are allegorical expressions of shattered hopes, but La Señora insists they are allusions to yet more black business and presses me to investigate.

'I feel the emotion,' she declares. 'Look at the eyes of these poor people. They are anxious to move their country forward. Also they need to broom these streets.'

Dutifully I make enquiries about the ghost train with Edgar, manager of the day in the hotel front office.

'I do not understand,' he replies. 'Please could you repeat the question in another form.'

I oblige and Edgar, giving a baffled shake of the head, consults Mariangela the receptionist. Fernando, the bored doorman-cum-waiter, joins the think-tank, followed by Fabiola who, sensing excitement, abandons her vacuum cleaner by the main entrance. Finally Carla the accountant, not to be excluded, freezes the guests' accounts and comes over from her computer to assist. They converse in low voices, glancing round in my direction from time to time. In due course Edgar returns to my end of the counter.

'Yes,' he nods, confirming La Señora's suspicions. 'It is true. We have a train. If you want the train you must wake up very early, but the journey is not so far, maybe ten hours.'

That's interesting, but not what I wanted to hear.

'Yes,' I say. 'But surely there should be *two* trains. Either someone sold the train or someone took the money and never bought the train. It was an *escándalo político*, *sí o no*?'

Fabiola returns to her vacuuming. She wants nothing of this. But Edgar, Carla, Mariangela and Fernando gaze first at me and then at each other. The furtive think-tank is reactivated. After a while, Edgar comes over.

'Yes,' he confirms, and then pauses, glancing round the deserted foyer. I lean forward across the counter. Edgar continues, dramatically. 'We had a President who took the train.'

'Ah! So that's it! He took the train! What happened next?'

'Nothing really. When he wanted to travel, he always took the train. Then at the end when he left, he left the train and took the car.'

'He took the car?'

'Yes. It was more convenient. Would you wish me to book you on the train to Rio Bamba? You can come back by bus. Or you can take the car.'

'Thank you, Edgar. I'll let you know. Perhaps I'll take the car. Like the President.'

I report back to La Señora.

'Exactly as I thought,' she confirms.

Changing tack, we visit the biggest private hospital in town and, after a successful meeting with the Director, lay the foundations for an affiliation with the Clinic, similar to plans for equally prestigious links to be forged in the United States,

243

Sweden and London, so that wherever our patients may chance to travel, medical cover will be assured, and vice versa on a reciprocal basis for patients of affiliated clinics when visiting Peru. La Señora sums things up succinctly.

'This is the most heavy part of our trip. But for these heavy moments we improve the future. Now more patients may be referred to the Clinic and we may look forward to receiving them.'

Then her attention is diverted.

'*¡Mira!*' she exclaims. 'Look! Observe that man there.' We look as directed. A dopey old man is up a ladder cleaning a sign. Whilst in Ecuador La Señora has been particularly strong on the allegorical and the mystical, with a keen sense of the primitive. It must be the influence of the timeless mountains and the enveloping forests. It is therefore no surprise when she continues in prophetic mood.

'The stairs are almost running down because he is not well support. He is doing his work very slow, looking round, forgetting where he is.' True. La Señora pauses for effect and then, whilst we wonder where she is taking us, concludes triumphantly. 'But he is working with *love*. We need to make the world part of our lives, rather than us being part of the world. I want you to think deeper what I am telling you. The world is falling down because of this.'

Perplexed, we nevertheless obediently set to work to extrapolate the parable for a better understanding of the good people of Ecuador. Maybe at this moment we have even stumbled on the very meaning of life itself. To assist us, La Señora continues.

'In these cases you may know that I have my imagination, my fantasy and my noble-ty. These are what I have.'

If only we could find the key to the conundrum then maybe it would explain why back at the hotel it takes Fernando, the doorman-cum-waiter, three trips to deliver a single cup of tea.

One to bring the steaming tea on the special collapsible table with the dying carnation in the pseudo-silver vase, one to check that everything is in order and to confirm that the tea is meeting with satisfaction and one to bring the necessary paperwork and to see if by chance I happen to have any loose change. We are spared from the unequal struggle when Wilson reminds us that time is running against us and that we have much to do before taking the evening flight back to Lima.

We hasten to collect La Señora's new antique furniture, the writing desk, the columns, a medley of chairs, the computerized games table for the husbands, plus a bronze-bound clothes chest that has somehow slipped in unnoticed.

'This ancient chest is of *roble*,' explains La Señora hurriedly, intercepting my eye and my thoughts simultaneously. 'Oak, you would say. It will last for ever. We will fill it with light linen and satin for the rocking cots and cradles of the newly arrived babies, scented with lavender of the very deepest blue and the petals of pink roses.'

As in Lima, the Quito process of payment is a ritual that cannot be abbreviated. In order that this may be so, no one concentrates on the business in hand. This enables La Señora to buy further impulsive items whilst a team of assistants descends on the pile of purchases armed with tape and cartons. Foremost amongst the new acquisitions is a sturdy couch with splayed claw-and-ball feet, suddenly vital to our needs, 'should anyone wish to recline unexpectedly'. There is now an urgent need to pass word to the Doctor to meet us with the big, once-white truck; nothing smaller will suffice to convey us from the airport. Especially with the guilty addition of an unknown number of paintings.

The contrary dry season further adds to our travails and once again the rain descends with increasing intensity, the grey mists swirl down the mountains and the city is enveloped in gloom.

'Now with this experience I am happy walking under the rain but I do not wish to queue for sightseeing under the rain,' declares La Señora.

There is nothing for it but to take refuge in a restaurant of repute to sample the finest Ecuadorian cuisine. Over the coffee we learn that the chef is Peruvian but by then such a minor detail is irrelevant. The moment of truth is upon us and with the stalwart help of Wilson we head for the airport. I count our pieces and note that they now tidily number a round dozen.

'Wilson,' says La Señora. Wilson is momentarily startled. I sense that even he had begun to forget his name. 'Wilson Sánchez, I wish to thank you for all your help.' So saying, La Señora presents the admirable Wilson with a bound memento of our visit accompanied by the four prancing horses. Wilson is visibly moved, as is La Señora, so I busy myself with the scales and the process of checking-in. The airline staff set to work with the baggage mountain, and the calculator, and deliver their verdict. Guilt is an expensive commodity.

'Oh!' exclaims La Señora, fumbling in her handbag for her purse. 'You know where is it? This delightful little Ecuadorian leather bag that I have bought has the magic to disappear all my things.'

Then, at my side one moment, she is gone the next, just like her purse, similarly disappearing. I reach into my pocket and do the necessary.

'Is our flight on time?' I enquire of the staff, for no particular reason other than wanting to know the answer.

'Oh, um, yes,' comes the response, 'as it happens, your plane may be a little late.'

'A little late?'

'Just an hour or so.'

'Where is it now? In the air, on the way?'

The check-in team confer. It's allowed by the rules. 'We will make an announce.'

La Señora reappears at my elbow. Uncanny. I start with the good news.

'The baggage is all through.'

'What baggage?'

'Now there is a problem with the flight.' I half expect her to ask 'What flight?'

'Oh,' she responds, both uninterested and disinterested, as though it is nothing to do with her, which in one way it isn't.

'The airport has been closed on account of the rain and fog,' I continue. 'The plane is either in Caracas or Bogotá, no one is sure which. Certainly it isn't here in Quito.'

Probably they forgot to radio the pilot to tell him that the rain had eased and our airport had reopened, so come on over. Probably he got fed up with sitting around in the cockpit in Caracas or Bogotá, parked the plane, fed the meter and even now was enjoying a bottle of *vino* with his girlfriend. Momentarily overlooking the fact that La Señora comes from a family with aviation in its veins, I suggest as much to her and immediately have cause to regret having given expression to such outrageous flights of my febrile fancy.

We say goodbye to Wilson again and we hope to see him again soon.

'I think we can wait comfortably if we go through,' I suggest.

'Oh, yes,' responds La Señora, brightening after the passing sadness of the leavetaking. 'I see lots of shops. Let me go see around. With my purse, who doesn't like to be alone.' With a swirl of mink she is gone.

The flight delay becomes significant. An unhappy depression of would-be passengers assembles, silent, submissive, resigned. La Señora, tour of the shops temporarily completed, explains the philosophy.

'These people they know how to dance before they get upset.'

Then she chats away, first here, then there. In no time she is

247

treating everyone to a presentation on the Clinic, complete with our life histories, receiving similar confidences in return. This activity exhausted, La Señora checks on the general state of nourishment amongst her new friends. The consensus is that everyone is hungry.

'What do you feel like?' questions La Señora. 'Lobsters? Steak?'

Rare? Well done? How about the wine list? But La Señora is serious and she scouts round to find a member of our airline. They are conspicuous by their absence; they've done the course, played before.

La Señora obtains sympathy from the security man on the hand-baggage machine but makes no real progress. Next, she tries a kiosk marked Aire Camarón, Air Shrimp, forgets the purpose of her enquiry and places an order for a box of Ecuadorian shrimps to accompany us to Lima ('The shrimps here are a little bit shrunk but we may try them'). Then her efforts are rewarded and she strikes gold.

'Follow me!' she directs the would-be passengers. 'We have a chicken supper.'

We follow. Some in hope, the more prescient trailing along out of idle curiosity. We wait. At length, instead of the chicken, a stringy uniformed lady of a certain age appears. She fixes me with a steely eye, beak tilted. How is it that all females are mind-readers in these latitudes? Without frills, she tells us that there will be no flight today and why not come back tomorrow? Pandemonium. I feel like an anthropologist studying behavioural patterns, until I remember that I too was supposed to be on that flight. La Señora is positive.

'Oh well,' she reflects carelessly. 'Better than crashing.'

'Yes, you can have your baggage back if you want,' promises the stringy official.

Have our baggage back! Perish the thought. Fortunately La Señora is not listening.

'What a shame,' I tell her. 'They won't give us our baggage back. Disgraceful.'

The following morning we set forth to seize the day and to turn the prolongation of our Quito visit to advantage. La Señora devises a scheme to export Ecuadorian leather goods to all quarters of the globe. Whilst setting this in motion we chance across a man with a cage full of ostriches. The leather scheme is abandoned and we gather the necessary details to enable the Doctor to run an ostrich farm on those scrubby hectares he tends south of Lima. We can call it the Hermogenes Abelardo Abasalon Ostrich Farm or something creative like that. La Señora says that adult ostriches can produce up to eighty little ostriches per year. Sounds like a gynaecologist's nightmare, but I expect the Doctor will cope. What with the high protein content of the meat and eggs big enough to feed a planeload of grounded passengers, plus the feathers, perfect for El Hipódromo Gold Cup days, I wonder why we never thought of it before. Out with the horses, out with the bulls, in with the birds. I also wonder how a group of framed ostriches will look on the intimate walls of the Doctor's consulting room in place of those handsome, happy matadors who can't believe their good fortune at hanging in such a strictly personal place, and how the patients will react to the change, if at all.

At last we have a moment to embark on a 'city tour' of Quito, hurrying into the hills to overlook the Ecuadorian capital from the vantage point of La Virgen del panecillo. Then down again to visit the ancient cathedral, Plaza Grande, Palacio de Carondelet and El Convento de San Francisco.

'The enchanted of these places you will never forget,' says La Señora. 'This moment will never repeat anymore and in this

Church of the Convent you will dignify your eyes just to look at these paints. These are some things that you will never pass the page. As much as you turn your face they will be in your deeper heart. The creators of these works of art had such affinity with the Bible that when they held it in their hands it pulsed with the warmth and life of a living creature. They lived in the physical universe of the Cosmos but they were encompassed by the spiritual universe of the Holy Scriptures.'

When we return to the hotel we learn that some of our fellow travellers have been enjoying their enforced stay in Quito not just for one day but for two, and that no aircraft from our selected airline has been sighted for forty-eight hours.

'Don't worry,' says Mauricio the liftman, cheerfully. 'It happens all the time.'

At the airport, the departure lounge assumes a reunion atmosphere. La Señora surveys the gathering.

'Well,' she reflects, 'really I don't see too much excitement here. Everyone is quite comfortable in the hotel.' She has been in touch with the Clinic. The Taxman has visited. '*Aaaay*,' she sighs heavily. 'No more shopping for a while.' She lapses into aggrieved silence at the injustice of it all. 'There's no point in returning to Lima. We should remain happy here.' Adding as an afterthought, 'The Bank can have the keys to the Clinic as a suppository.' And she wills the aircraft not to appear.

But not all wishes are granted. In Lima, Dr Hermogenes greets us with the faithful, big, once-white truck. Customs delay us for a moment or two as we wheel four heavily laden baggage carts past their startled gaze. I explain what we have: an unknown number of paintings and a quantity of furniture and if there is any problem please keep everything because we are tired and need to go to bed. That settles it, we receive the accolade of the green nod and we set about loading the truck. As we do so, two tourists in safari suits appear without their rucksacks.

'Would you believe it?' they protest, nonplussed. 'There was no room for them on the aircraft.'

Driving back to the Clinic the Doctor gives us the latest news.

'Nothing has changed so much,' he tells us. 'It is like the same woman in different knickers.' La Señora looks at him sharply. 'Yes,' he confirms hurriedly, 'we had some rain. Nothing much, it was just the small sort of rain that bothers.'

No sooner are we back in the Clinic than Aunt Gertrudis is ringing to admonish La Señora for her extravagance in journeying to Ecuador, and for abandoning the helm of our fragile enterprise at such a critical moment.

'We undertook investment, marketing and professional development,' declares La Señora with admirable conviction, thereby reaffirming that travelling needs no justification, least of all in South America.

Whereupon Aunt Gertrudis is forced to reveal her hand. 'Well,' she pleads, 'next time you go anywhere, please be certain to invite me with you.'

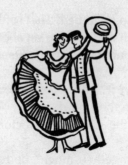

20

'Lima la Gris'

Life is grey. We are grey. Lima is grey. The cheerless mists of the Limeño winter were not for the sun-loving Incas. The conquistadors were deceived into building their capital at the mouth of the River Rimac, the 'talking river' in Quechua, now but a turgid trickle in place of those long-forgotten dancing waters that gurgled and sang as they raced over the river bed boulders. 'You may think you have won,' said the Incas softly. 'But you and your kind will suffer the gloom of eternal shade. May the dark and joyless clouds rest forever on your treacherous and arrogant heads.' Now the once fertile plains are buried under the urban sprawl of the vast city, home to more than one third of Peruvians. And suffer we do, the sunshine deprivation syndrome, even though *los Limeños* affect to be untroubled by the climate.

'Yes, it is cloudy,' observes La Señora philosophically. 'The sun went off. Let the sun come when he wants. Then Peru will be smiling and the world will smile with us. We must have sunshine in our lives, even if it is not in the sky.'

252

Be that as it may, 'Lima the Grey', sad city of black business, black money and grey mist, no more the 'Pearl of the Pacific', reflects our mood. The winter weather is dominating our spirits and the Bank is governing our pockets. Even La Señora has to acknowledge the prevailing difficulties.

'Now at this time we are not in a spending moment,' she declares, arranging and setting out her new Ecuadorian furniture, consigning the davenport to Leonardo for the necessary renovations and having some difficulty, not entirely unforeseen, with siting the Corinthian columns. 'The situation for our possible loan, some of which as you know I have already invested, is still in suspense. I cannot reveal more, except that we are in a savings moment. In fact, we need to go in reversal. I know how to do this. When I was young they called me the penny keeper.'

For an instant I sense that the Doctor is on the point of asking for that to be put in writing, but he is forestalled.

'I am very pain full,' continues the orator, collapsing dramatically on to the new and conveniently handy reclining couch with the splayed feet, 'and the situation tries to flat me down. It is the Bank that is boring on us.' Pause for thought. 'But I am not the kind of ship that I am sunk.' Respectful silence. 'Now I am on the horse, I am going to revolutionary the situation in my Clinic. With my two little fingers I can move the world and in the Bank I will dot the eyes. I am preparated for this moment. With all the influences I have, I am the head of the mouse but not the tail of the lion.'

'This is very baroque language you are using,' remarks the Doctor, and then wishes that he hadn't. There are some people in this world who should never be crossed.

La Señora chooses to ignore the interruption, for the moment at least. 'In this executive conversation we are working on our future,' she concludes. 'Before I did not have great knowledgement of these matters. Now I do and I know that you are not successful until you are.'

It is left to the profundity of the ensuing silence to match the profundity of the sentiment. There are no further interruptions.

We start by engaging a new accountant; our tax return would undoubtedly benefit from a touch of lateral creativity. Señor Melquiades is immensely keen, well qualified and anxious to do everything on time, maybe even ahead of time but sadly, he is impetuous.

'So how do you manage the expenses?' he enquires, reasonably enough. 'Or is it as I think, total anarchy?'

¡Caramba! ¡Hombre! Now we need another accountant; staff turnover, that's what it's called. La Señora moves ever forward. She has a bevy of cards up her sleeve, ranging from herbal medicine to hi-tech.

'I am feeding the people free coffee all the day,' she confides. Maybe the sale of *uña de gato*, *maca* from the high Andes and the secret potions of *la selva* will follow close behind. 'See now how much faster they are running. They will finish their work in a wink.'

Thus advised, I observe, expecting to see demented Lupi Pancho, the wiry electrician, and mop-haired Leonardo da Painter functioning like men with six arms. I don't say anything dampening to La Señora, but there is no discernible difference in their vacant behaviour, no change from the normal imperceptible speed of advance. Slow ahead both engines at best, one pace forward and two paces back after lunch. The fax machine remains wedded to the front door entry-phone and the water-heater resolutely declines to influence the tepid shower. As for Leonardo, he obviously sees revarnishing the new furniture as a pensionable occupation and is determined that no amount of caffeine will affect his non-productivity. Overdosing energetic Ernestina with coffee has adverse effects and she becomes apathetically, unaccountably lackadaisical, her lethargic ledgers lying open but neglected on her desk, whilst striding Señorita Hilda, brooking no substitutes, is resolutely immune to alternative therapies.

Moving from the *cafetería* coffee to the under-utilized overabused Clinic computers, from nutrition to technology, La Señora engages a practical man, Jeremias, to link the screens into an information web in the fashionable mode. Patient data base, last appointment, next visit, password-protected treatment information, pharmacy action, laboratory follow-up, billing, payments. Basic. Except that we have to engage a second practical man, Humberto Campodonico, to sort it out and to make it work.

'The problem is that now we have the new computers in a net, we have a mist up of things,' comments La Señora. 'I am quite despaired because of the inexperience of these machines, perhaps we are suffering from an electrical short cut. All you have to do is to pull the string of the telephone and pass it to the internet. Sorry for talking science. I am not a scientific. I am just a regular human being.' Interval for breath. 'Poor Jeremias,' she adds gratuitously, referring to the first practical man and launching into another of her recurring themes, principally for my benefit. 'Before this he was a military. So there is confusion in his mind and Humberto must unassemble everything before our eyes.'

Humberto Campodonico, rare genius that he is, cuts the mustard. Then, as an encore, he turns his attentions unnecessarily to the Clinic's closed circuit video system. This is functioning perfectly satisfactorily, theoretically enabling the progress of day-surgery conducted by Dr Hermogenes and Dr Cleeber in the increasingly busy operating theatre to be screened to select audiences of yet-to-be-invited senior medical professionals in the auditorium. Nevertheless, Humberto dismantles and reassembles the equipment, dusts around and flaps about in the mysterious manner of his occult trade and then charges what he considers to be an appropriate fee for the service.

At least we fare better with the video than with the Clinic washing machine. The man from the mountains, self-declared technician, arrives to effect repairs, randomly wields his rusty spanner and hi-tech clanging hammer, spends a morning arranging the individual components artistically on the laundry floor and then vanishes, defeated by the mechanical complexity of the twenty-first century, thereby seriously jeopardizing the supply of white coats within the Clinic and occasioning a dearth of starched lace caps for Nurses Dulce and Dolores. Thus we ambiguously advance: a stream of people coming in to fix things and a stream of money going out to pay for their uncertain services.

The shelves of our embryonic medical library, housed on the balcony surrounding the auditorium, are gradually filling with learned tomes. The project has been affected alternately by the euphoria engendered by the possibility of improved refinancing schemes and by periodic spending freezes. Nevertheless, progress is being made, albeit intermittently. To accommodate La Señora's personal tastes, there are also generous sections on art and horticulture and she devotes considerable time to arranging and cataloguing the archives, punctuated with calls for assistance with the top shelf.

'Help me with this please,' she cries, 'I am not so tall. I am trying to put the things in order in an economical way but I am short handed, I cannot paint the stars in the sky and off the steps I keep slippering down.' And then she adds quickly, in case we should be under any misapprehension, 'But know that the smallest are the ones that will last the longest and know also that I have good knees since a child, I can bend and come. Although at last I am glad to sit; I have a little tired in my back.' It is a reminder that we must harness the energy whilst the enthusiasm endures.

We review our marketing strategy yet again and enrol the Clinic as a 'provider' with the leading Peruvian healthcare insurance schemes, both endeavours reaping no noticeable return. In the evenings, La Señora delivers compellingly innovative prenatal classes to a full circle of intent shadowy faces illuminated by candlelight in the darkened auditorium, exploring the miracles of conception and birth to the accompaniment of the soothing sound of water flowing over the adjacent *catarata*, previously our waterfall-without-water but now replete.

'You are pregnant too,' La Señora tells the accompanying husbands, breaking the spell. 'Now you must learn to change and bathe the baby.'

The bashful husbands blink. It is a new concept for the medallion men.

Our ground-breaking Clinic is synonymous with new concepts. Shiny, colourful posters are prepared giving notice of the inaugural Seminar to be conducted by no less than John M. Lane himself of The John M. Lane Institute of Hospital and Clinic Administration, 200 copies to be distributed throughout Lima. The cost of recorded delivery is not inconsiderable but the return will make it worthwhile. Then Dr Hermogenes, embarking on a personal initiative, hits on a well-intentioned alternative and more economical system of distribution, engaging an unknown taxi driver, supposedly an acquaintance of Abraham, to do the job at a fraction of the cost.

Interestingly, but not unfathomably, the prestigious not-to-be-missed inaugural one-day Seminar of the newly formed august Institute is attended by an audience of six students and four nuns. The number of participants is swollen to a grand total of eleven by the late arrival of Aunt Gertrudis, who then sleeps through the entire proceedings, awakening only for the buffet lunch and a glass or two of chilled Tacama.

The translation of John M. Lane's off-the-wall words of wisdom from the podium into Castellano is obligingly undertaken by Medical Student One. He freely adds to the text as he sees fit and helpfully answers all questions without reference to the Chair. 'The golden rule in business,' he tells the audience, with infinite sagacity, commendable in one so young, 'is always be sure to use other people's money.'

After such an unprecedented flush of excitements and developments, La Señora is in need of a change of scene.

'I started my classes well, but I don't think I like doing any more here in this moment. Now I am leaving to organize my closet,' she declares. 'That will organize my life. Excuse me for this day. Maybe tomorrow I better don't come.'

That will be a relief. The geography of my accommodation, with its balcony overlooking the heavily booked auditorium, has meant that in recent weeks I have been unexpectedly finding myself on occasion something of an inadvertent intruder in the gush of newly scheduled and at times unannounced activities, leaping innocently from my bed only to realize too late that I am centre stage in one of Dr Vonday's early morning menopausal lectures (as thinly attended as an inaugural seminar) or featuring as star turn in the senior keep-fit class conducted by Statuesque Wellington Fisher, newly head-hunted from *gimnasio* Body 2000.

Whilst our beautiful Healthcare Clinic has become the talk of the town, certainly amongst the ladies, a conspiracy of silence hangs over the subject of the national economy, deep in depression and one of the keys to our survival. The non-existent world recession is given the blame and the Press is fed with false statistics. Growth indices are multiplied, unemployment figures are divided. Simple arithmetic. There is no debate, no reinflationary measures are taken. A lowering of interest levels would be a good starting point but the vested interests are too many. This is a place of dark currents. Perhaps the problem will drift away, like an uninvited guest. Whatever happens, it will be too late for many businesses and enterprises. The question remains: can we ourselves continue? Or maybe we should climb on the bandwagon and open a Bank.

I am drawn to one side over cocktails.

'Maybe you are not understanding, señor, *sí o no*?'

'*Sí*. Maybe not.'

'Why is it that here in Peru, home of the potato and growers of rice, we are importing potatoes and rice?'

'It does seem a bit strange.'

'It is not strange. It is commission. Destroy the internal economy, import more, more commission for the pocket. Easy. Naturally, something similar is going along with the arms imports and the narco-traffic, the Colombian marching powder, call it what you will.'

'Cut the cake three ways?'

'*Exacto*. Now you are learning. The politicians, the armed forces, the shadowy secret friends. Maybe it is not your way, heh? Think for always of *coimas* and *subornos*. Commissions and inducements. This will help your knowledgement. In things such as these we are not a country. People are living around here but we have no direction, no economic unity or purpose.'

'The President is making some changes in the Cabinet. Maybe that will help?'

'No, my friend. They are just changing the flies on the cake. We need to change the cake.'

The unravelling of disintegrating society. More poverty, more unemployment. Less education. More street crime; more robberies; more assaults; more kidnappings; more fraud; more dishonesty. The law of the urban jungle.

'And if here we are conversing historically, reflect on the

legacy of Pearl Harbor, Hiroshima and Nagasaki. Now you are understanding better, *sí* señor?'

Eh? 'Yes. Thank you.' No, not really. I am just hearing the words, an innocent abroad.

La Señora is herself victim of an assault outside Casa Bonomini. Six o'clock in the evening, dusk, returning from shopping and her bag is stolen, ripped from her grasp as she is knocked to the ground and dragged along the pavement. Her arm is broken in the ferocity of the attack. The target of previous thefts and assaults in Lima, she is resilient and philosophical as she describes what happened.

'This is a dangerous country, you can call it. The robber, he was a nice boy with well appearance. He was ashamed of what he was doing. He was looking to me, his eyes saying "I'm sorry", but suddenly in the moment that I am entering the house he pulled my bag very strong and I fell because of the power he had on me. My heart jumped out and I shrank. I called to the guard but he was too away. I am tired to be stolen. How do you feel to be robberied? I am wounded in my broken soul as well as in my broken bone. I cannot say too many big things on this subject. With my arm in plaster now I am incapable of my everything. You all have two wings but now I have only one. I am lost. However, my arm is only one and hopefully in the future it will work again very fine but I wonder who is the source of these attacks? I am not going to cry for this. At this moment it is not convenient for me to get excited. Just know that from now on I shall be learning how to shoot. You knew that? Well, now you may know it better.'

One thing appears certain. The dream of defeated presidential candidate El Cholo of having an electoral replay seems forlorn.

'I don't feel him too happy,' observes the Doctor wisely. 'But let us see. In this country you must remember that those things that look certain are sometimes the most uncertain.'

I nod in acquiescence, neither of us appreciating the verity of this delphic prognostication, which has but a short time to fulfilment.

The relevant international bodies return to Lima one by one to shake their heads and to wag their fingers at El Chino, President for an unconstitutional third term, but they are toothless tigers. Some are not even granted space in the presidential agenda; the disdainful diary is very full. Anyway, these officials have families to feed, they need to safeguard their lucrative positions. Rumour has it that the national intelligence service, the appropriately abbreviated SIN, holds secret film of the leading players engaged in unfortunate indiscretions in darkened rooms on previous visits to Peru. Along with a reputed further twenty thousand incriminating videos for use as convenient against public figures and any other targets who might mistakenly consider stepping out of line.

'So, what of Señor Montesinos?' I ask the well-informed Doctor, whose consultations with his patients are invariably sociably wide-ranging.

'Ah, the shadowy power behind the throne? Well, in terms of corruption, Señor Montesinos is much better at it than the others, that is the difference. Now they are all very upset to discover that he has taken more than his fair share of the pickings. One day it may dawn on someone that the heart of the problem is our constitution. It would be simpler to change that, rather than waiting in vain for the flawed theory of evolution to effect a change in human nature. We need to protect the ideals of government from human inadequacy.'

'I have a theory,' says Medical Student One, keen as always to share his ideas. 'Well, I read it actually. Have you noticed that polling booths look like French urinals and that the ballot boxes always look like old grocery cartons and that the voters can never get their ballot papers into the box because they are smiling at the camera and not paying attention? This is what we need to reform. It needs to be less prosaic. That's what the book says. For example, you could have lasers, computerized coloured fountains, music and flashing lights, the voters revolving in giant cylinders caught by centrifugal forces, assault courses for famous people, musical ballot boxes, games of skill and chance, lucky numbers, prizes and forfeits, voters abseiling from hovering helicopters on to ballot beds, with naked maidens romping mistily in a flurrying fog of floating votes, a sort of hyperactive political bubble bath. Everything. A jamboree. I have been reading about this quite a lot, actually. It needs modernizing and popularizing.'

'What about maintaining the dignity of the day?'

'Well, yes. You could do that too.'

Clearly La Señora's pioneering foray in her clown's outfit was merely the first step; the rest will surely follow.

Our unaccustomed burst of activity in the Clinic has led to an overdose of solemnity.

'Have patience. The less you seek the hare, the sooner it jumps,' Dr Hermogenes reminds us sagely, philosopher par excellence. He is right. Our salvation is in the lap of the gods. Or in frustratingly silent Arequipa, yet to pronounce on our much-needed loan.

Perhaps I should seek out my old friend, the miracle man of *La Pamplonada*. Meanwhile, we have other diversions.

I enquire after the Doctor's horses. We have not been to the races for some time and there has even been talk of a sale.

'We are in a quiet moment,' he tells me. 'Unfortunately, Expectativa put her foot in a hole and that was the end. Then Rescate decided not to be a runner any more and is near the end. And Big Bertha we sold for a good price. Except the money is still on the way. In a short time we should have two new horses to run, Hacker and Espatano. That is an Egyptian name or even a Greek. Not Hacker, the other. Anyway, both are very fast.'

'Ah. And Mickey Moto?'

'Now he is back from Miami.'

'With er . . . ?

'¡Sí! Definitivamente.'

With recollections of Mrs Moto's appealing skirts, La Señora has driven the sport of kings underground. The Doctor's mobile phone rings.

'It is the Japonezee,' hisses La Señora. 'When he doesn't say the name, it is him.'

She weakens to the extent that one lunchtime we drive downtown to visit the long-established Maury Hotel, where in the Dardanus Bar the eponymous Peruvian winner of the Classic South American sprint race was historically ridden to the counter to partake of a silver pail of pisco sour. With his prodigious memory, the Doctor recalls that the colourful celebration occurred forty years ago, whilst La Señora studies the commemorative photographs and rules that the fashions belong to a slightly earlier era. But both are in complete accord on one point.

'Here in Peru in those days there were a lot of chatting people. Antique people. Elegant professionals with shorts and time to spare.'

A nostalgic silence follows in memory of those not so distant but gone for ever feudal times.

The Doctor has horses, I have courses. Enthusiasm for further seminars at the John M. Lane Institute having temporarily waned, I enrol instead in *bailando tropical* classes to hone my Latina Americana and salsa dancing techniques, plus a touch of Amazonic *tecnocumbia*, or more correctly, *tropicumbia*, in anticipation of forthcoming never-to-be-received invitations. Encouraged by modest success, I add *La Marinera* to the repertoire; only in Peru could a *Marinera* dancer be seen taking a mobile telephone call in mid-pirouette. There is just one setback. After months of preparation, I am expelled from my group on the very eve of our end-of-term presentation and relegated to the audience to sit alongside the watchful assembly of proud parents. My public participation in the graceful dance of love from northern Peru must wait for another day. It's not my fault that my parents couldn't make it.

The spirit of self-improvement knows no bounds and I return to the classroom in a final thrust for mastery of the elusive Spanish tongue, the key to understanding the heart, soul and pulse of Peru. And to giving unimpeded seminars. As it happens, the college classrooms are full of earnest Chinese, their inscrutable sense of humour as grey as a Limeño day. If these people have poetry in their hearts and music in their lives, then it is a well-kept secret. A hundred and fifty years ago, the first one hundred and fifty Chinese arrived in Peru. Now they number one in ten of the population. Chinatown in Lima thrives and no one wishes to contemplate the future too closely.

The time for Plaza de Acho is not yet on us, but out in the provinces, up in the *sierra*, the new season is stirring. Antonio the Mexican matador is in town and La Señora needs no second bidding to stage one of her famous dinner parties.

'This dinner is a special situation,' she informs us. 'We shall be eating the mothers of the Mexican bulls.' Whilst we digest the significance of this, La Señora moves the conversation along with a semi-non-sequitur. 'Just now Antonio had a bullfight horn in the leg, but really he is fine.'

I observe. Yes, Antonio looks quite fine. We toreadors are made of stern stuff. Antonio is enjoying the Doctor's pisco sours, traditional curtain-raiser to Peruvian feasts. The Doctor shares his *receta secreta*. His time as a medical student was well spent.

'To three parts of the white spirit of the grapes, distilled in such a way that the *conquistadores* knew, is added one part the squeeze of the lemons and one part the plain syrup, not forgetting the white, whisked, of an egg. Nothing more except this sprinkle of cinnamon and these drops of angostura. The name comes from the town of Pisco of course, on *el río* Pisco, two hundred kilometres south of Lima in the province of Ica. You will meet with impostors but remember that the true pisco comes only from Peru.'

So saying, the Doctor hands round brimming glasses of the frothy, freshly blended elixir, as smooth as satin.

'Maybe it is too fierce for your flavour?' enquires La Señora, anxiously. 'Pisco is Peru and it should be not too much and not too less. At all times it should be extremely excellent.'

Pisco should really be a Peruvian unit of time.

'Hallo! Have you been waiting long?'

'Well, three and a half piscos actually.'

'Oh my goodness! I *am* sorry. Fancy another?'

Much more precise than the elastic *un ratito*, 'just a moment', which can extend for anything up to half an hour and even beyond, particularly when you imagine you are in a hurry.

There is no seating plan for the famously eccentric dinners, no *placement*. Sit where you fall. Sometimes it is a case of musical chairs; so difficult to remember who has been invited. Often the meal is not ready much before midnight.

'Now they are informing me that they are prepared,' announces La Señora, calmly oblivious to the passage of time. 'Start everyone, I am putting the seat on the pot. And by the way, I am sorry for the amount of this soup. The cook she prepared it in just the large size.'

For the bullfighter's dinner the silver platters come and go and then, unexpectedly, there is a lull in proceedings. The menu has come to a halt, there is no *postre*, no pudding, no more food, no anything. La Señora must have been distracted during the planning process. Abraham the artilleryman saves the situation. In his masquerading butler's coat he circumnavigates the table, taking careful aim and solemnly laying a bar of chocolate on the expectant fine bone china before each guest. The conversation hardly flickers; La Señora's dinner parties are famously famous and deservedly so.

On to the brandy, to the tequila and salt. Antonio presents his host with a box of Cuban cigars. He has taken heed of La Señora's oft-stressed stipulation that 'the guest should always bring something to the house, even if it is just a smile'. The Doctor is pleased, the cigars are his favourites.

'Just a few puffs,' he advises us joyfully through a cloud of smoke as opaque as a Limeño winter's day. 'It is enough.'

'Rolled on the inside thigh of a young virgin,' Antonio informs us authoritatively, emboldened by the tequila. The more sheltered amongst us blush at the mere mention of such heavenly happenings. La Señora gives a forgiving flourish of her longer-than-long Greta Garbo cigarette holder, blows smoke into the chandelier and ignores the indiscretion, talking through the momentary quickening of the pulses.

'In my deep,' she tells us, 'I like to touch the persons who I have next to me. My husband Dr Hermogenes says "Don't touch the people when you talk". But still I have the problem and maybe I will divorce because of this and because I talk too loud. It is a problem of the volcano Misti, one day I start with the left foot and some days with the right. But we will not talk to that whilst we are having dinner. One pleasure is that, the other is the other. No mixing.'

Antonio the bullfighter is sitting next to La Señora, following her conversation attentively, or at least trying hard. He sips his provocative tequila.

'You are a large woman,' he pronounces after some thought, stroking her arm.

'Do not touch my rounds please,' says La Señora, turning sharply. 'I am a private person and I do not know you too much.'

'Large in the heart,' clarifies the gallant matador, somewhat hastily and firmly crossing his arms.

La Señora leads her life forwards. There are very few yesterdays for her, except just occasionally after the famous dinner parties.

'For me the evening was too much. This morning when I appear my eyes out of the duvet, I try to get up but back down goes my head. I was in a full depression in my bed. I think my soul went away for a while and I am like in a boat now. Of course, I am taking tablets but I think these pills are making me adverse. Look, perhaps I am drinking the pills for sleeping by mistake or perhaps I am truly sick. In fact, I took so many pills and tablets there is confusion in my *estómago*. Today I am a conflict person. You can see me slippering off this chair and maybe I am contaging the people with germs. I am thirsty, I need a deep glass. Today my body hurts of the wine. It was Greek wine. Those Greeks, they are too bad. I am sure I am feeling better tomorrow but that is by the by. Now we must go to San Bartolo. It is the feast of Saint Peter and Saint Paul.'

'Surely not? I mean, I know it is, but couldn't we perhaps, um, rest a little today?'

It is as though I hadn't even spoken.

'We must leave immediately. Everything has been prepared with such excitement, we cannot be a disappointment to them. It is a national fiesta, the party will be for all the family. We may drink a lot and distant Cousin Antenogenes, whom you have not met, will put fireworks on the ocean.'

Accordingly, we all go south to the diminutive fishing village of San Bartolo, where fortuitously Cousin Antenogenes owns an out-of-season seasonal hotel.

'He is the owner,' I am told. 'He is running as his wish. It is ours for the day.'

The fishermen's annual parade of San Pedro is keeping *la hora Señora*, so we are just in time. The procession winds its way along the seafront, followed more or less sonorously by the village brass band, the music for each player clipped to the collar of the man in front.

'Some of these people in the band,' I am advised, 'they are policemans.'

'This ceremony,' I enquire, 'is to say *gracias* or *por favor*?'

Cousin Antenogenes considers. 'Both,' he confirms. 'The fishermen are grateful for what they had and they are hoping for more.'

We enjoy lunch on the hotel terrace, warmly wrapped against the cool of the wind; those eternal Pacific rollers easing themselves through the narrow harbour mouth and exploding against the rocks below us in a thunder of white foam.

'From sitting here we see all the panorama from the table,' observes La Señora comfortably. 'How important is the good view.'

It is time for the statue of Saint Peter to go afloat with the fishermen. There is a complication. Peru is about to play Ecuador at football and the harvesters of the sea are unwilling to miss a moment of the promised spectacle. It's a difficult case of divided loyalties.

'The breeze is making blow and they say the sea is too crispy,' explains the Doctor.

Good order finally prevails and off go the reluctant fishers to do their duty whilst the rest of us settle down for the big match.

Tradition dictates that the fishing boats have to stay out on the waters until the first fish is caught; the indications are that this won't take too long today. Probably just a tiddler is all that is needed and with luck they should be back before half-time.

Medical Students One and Two are disgruntled travellers to San Bartolo, but La Señora's word is law. Medical Student One has invited his friends to watch the football on the big screen at Casa Bonomini and even as we partake of sustaining Mari-Vis, or *pelotazos*, that barbaric mix of whisky and Coca-Cola, the would-be invitees are gathered despairingly at the gates of the big house, robbed of the opportunity to participate in the anticipated feast of goals. Similar happenings have occurred previously with La Señora's lunch parties. It is not my turn to speak but I must check later with the Doctor to see if this is a hereditary condition on the mother's side.

Now there is an additional complication. *Los aficionados* adjudge the television screen of El Hotel Los Delfines to be too small for such an important occasion. Cousin Antenogenes is quick to quell unrest in the crowd and makes amends by setting up a second set of the same size alongside the first so that we may watch proceedings in duplicate, in visionary stereo. He need hardly have bothered, and those anxious fishermen, back on shore in record time, could have tended their tranquil nets the entire afternoon to better purpose. Ecuador score first one goal and then another.

'What is the situation in this game?' enquires La Señora.

'Tía Coraima,' chorus the family. '*¡Por favor!* Aunt Coraima, please pay attention!'

'I am totally concentrate,' protests La Señora. 'This game is entirely comprehensive for me. I just need to know who to how. How to who?'

'You mean what is the score? Now we are losing by two goals,' replies the Doctor sadly.

'Well, my forecast was that we would lose by three. We have

a political problem here, it is a political matter. And a question of national personality. Sorry that I have to tell you that.'

'I am not offended,' says the Doctor. 'I have free press in my mind.'

'I think soon it will arrive to seven goals,' observes Cousin Antenogenes cheerfully.

Suddenly, Peru pull one goal back. The whole of San Bartolo erupts with passion. The Doctor is pleased to remind us of a different scene during a World Cup match.

'When the English score the goal, I see Prince Charles he just rise the hand. British phlegm, heh?'

Regrettably there are no more goals for Peru today. Medical Student One shrugs.

'We lost the match. Now again I am making stiff the upper lip.' It has become his mantra.

True to form, the disappointing outcome of the game is soon forgotten.

'Now the musicians they will make a serenade,' comments Cousin Antenogenes. 'If it is good we can jump on the tables to applause them.'

Rockets explode high above the harbour to mark the successful conclusion of the piscatorial part of the proceedings, glasses are refilled and the extended family circle draws tight to conduct their biannual review of matters outstanding. Is it the empty glasses or the empty lives that have to be refilled?

'For them,' clarifies La Señora, 'if there is no TV for watching, the life is dead. They should be looking to their own lives, not looking to others.'

Eavesdroppers never hear well of themselves, but the excellent acoustics of the Dolphin Hotel defeat me. Cousin Antenogenes should hold orchestral concerts on the terrace during the summer months, the soft waves lapping on the shore, the balmy evening air. But for the moment, the family elders get down to business. Reception is loud and clear. 'Aunt

Abundia lost her earrings in the desert . . . maybe the butler ate them . . . as for the other, you will see that his weight is rising . . . when you have a mistress you must eat in two houses.' Above the noise of the breaking waves and exploding fireworks comes the predictable enquiry. 'But how can he be watering the broccoli if he won a prize for being a ballerina?'

Eavesdroppers, even the inadvertent, never hear well of themselves.

On our way back to Lima from San Bartolo, La Señora is in a reflective mood.

'Fireworks they always fill me with sparkling emotions,' she comments. 'But those with not so much family and no cousins, how do they manage for gossipings and fightings?'

In spite of our efforts to the contrary and the surge of innovations at the Clinic, in spite of fiestas, dinner parties, dancing, horses and other distractions, little by little grey Lima, black politics, the ill-managed economic recession, the yawning Bank and the vicious mugging all conspire to take their toll of La Señora's customary irrepressibly ebullient optimism. Maybe she is indeed suffering from sunshine deprivation; possibly the malaise is more fundamental. It is good to have money, so they say, if only for financial reasons.

'These people they throw the stones and hide the hand,' says La Señora. 'My tears are exhausted of crying. I am sitting in a reality I cannot recognize. We need to talk and think. Everything needs to be chop-ped.' She surveys the financial statements arrayed on her desk. 'Look, all my life is distributed on little bits of paper. I do not wish to be a person in the red. I wish to be in the blue, to share the luxurious happiness of the clouds dreaming in the sky, to enjoy my lostness, to have my heart very good and to taste the feel of freedom. I do not want to mark my life by lines, I like to see the ducks flying on the wing in the horizon and to watch the stars shining in the night. Dr Hermogenes is right. We must be patient and wait for the rabbit. Let us go in search of soft winter warmth and seek gentle zephyrs to caress away our cares. I see myself so pale as a mashed potato or even a cold pork. I need to seek sun and stimulation.'

At this declaration, passing Señorita Hilda freezes in mid-stride and turns to gaze in disapproving disbelief at the speaker. The point is made but La Señora affects to be un-deterred.

'As we are in the southern hemisphere,' she continues airily, scarcely faltering, 'we must go northwards, for example, we could return to Chiclayo, where, says the guide book, travellers may greet the antiquities and wonders of the pre-Hispanic ancient civilizations and a flight of six hundred kilometres will bring us to sugar cane, rice and cotton plantations (not to mention derelict haciendas and defunct steam engines that once served these great plantations), previously the centre of the Mochica culture before the rule of the Chimu, to visit El Museo Bruning at Lambayeque and the Valley of the Pyramids at Tucume, concluding the day amidst *los artesanos* in the nearby town of Monsefu when saturated with history to buy baskets and carvings from the local craftsmen.'

'Do you think this is the moment to leave the Clinic?' I query, cautiously.

'Listen, there is more in the book. We can see the tomb of El Señor de Sipan and the coastal villages of Pimentel and Santa Rosa, with their traditional *caballitos de totora* used by the fishermen, the 'reed horses' of the ocean. In Pimentel there is the former home of Peruvian Air Force hero Capitán José Quinones, contemporary of my father, who lost his life in action against Ecuador in 1941. You are interested in these

272

things and he is commemorated on our ten-soles banknotes, although really he should have been given a higher denomination. I don't know who decides these things.'

Señorita Hilda sniffs, puffs out her nicely rounded downy cheeks, shakes her head, turns and leaves. But La Señora is determined to finish.

'After seeing the vast adobe fortress of Chan Chan, capital of the Chimu culture which succeeded that of the Mochica, as previously indicated, with their mystical Sun and Moon Temples, we may move to the mellifluously named Trujillo, "land of eternal spring" and city of lace-barred windows and intricately carved balconies, three hours by bus. Relatively unvisited and uncrowded compared to Machu Picchu, the sense of history and antiquity is more all-pervading at Chan Chan, finally abandoned to the Incas in the middle of the fifteenth century.' La Señora closes the book. 'Just think,' she reflects, 'no windows, no doors, no keys. The free life. They didn't care about money, they didn't care about nothing. *Sí o no*? Give time to the time, time to think. I remember we have been briefly to Trujillo before, but then the work was so hard with no opportunity to be tourists.'

However, even the Doctor demurs. Enough is enough.

'No. This is not the time to travel, better to think here in the Clinic,' he says firmly.

La Señora looks at him in surprise. Then she pronounces, turning in my direction.

'Although you would like to travel again, especially as Trujillo is the home of the *Marinera* dance and centre for *el caballo de paso*, the Peruvian pacing horse, this journey must be postponed to another more suitable day. The Mochica and Chimu civilizations are reminders of our inheritance and I read recently that "against the depth and breadth of this cultural tapestry, the itinerant aberrations and irritations of contemporary Peru fall into perspective" and that "the fabric of the

heritage will withstand the stresses of the current disarray".
This confirms to me that our Clinic, as a microcosmic element
of the whole, can surely survive. *Sí o no*?'

'That means you are expecting good news from Arequipa at
any moment?'

'I cannot say just now. My cellular may ring and interrupt
our conversation, disappointing you.'

It is the Bank that unwittingly confirms the advent of the long-
awaited good tidings. Aided and abetted by his colleagues, our
banker, proud possessor of the nice frame surrounding La
Señora's epic portrait of The Tortured Nude, devises yet
another refinancing package and then advises that the charge
for this doubtful service will be a further fifteen thousand
dollars. But they have finally overplayed their hand.

'I spotted them,' La Señora tells me afterwards, 'I saw them
clink the eyes.'

Accordingly, she apprises them of her thoughts, propelled
by new-found confidence and sure in the knowledge that she
is about to dispense with their ruinous support.

'Normally I can put so much flowers in my mouth when I
talk to them, I don't speak with pumpkins on the tongue unless
I can blow the golden carriages but not this time. I am not a
rude person on this but now they are very resented and totally
disinflado,' she informs us happily. 'Out of air.' Even deflated.

'Oh! Sorry!' say the grey men. 'Our calculator slipped. The
commission should be only half that price.'

Commission? La Señora doesn't bother to reinflate the
bankers. Like limp balloons on the morning after, they have
had their time.

'For them, even my company is not so welcome now,' says
La Señora, with the careless relish of someone free of financial
shackles for the first time in many months. 'Oh, they are just
inexpensive persons, they are so cheap in feelings,' she con-

cludes. 'Believe me, normally I forget in ten minutes but with these people I remember a long time. Now I have rung them and stopped the situation. I told them: "Don't call me hallo for anything. The advice you are giving to me I invert it to you. Please get back out of my life."'

'Wonderful words. I think we got the loan, *sí o no*?'

'This is Peru. Do you remember those fighting bulls we watched in the shadow of majestic Misti, the volcano? Well, all I can tell you is that all the heaving and struggling – monolithic, yes? – is now in the past. From today the Clinic will soar ever upwards, like the condors of the Colca Canyon. And soon we may open health centres for the poor.'

¡Bravo! At last we have the loan! *Mamasita linda* indeed!

On the political front, defeated El Cholo stages a grand demonstration against victorious El Chino. As a result of the historically named *La Marcha de los Cuatro Suyos*, taking its title from the four provinces of the great Inca Empire, Lima is paralysed by riots for a day. Then the crowds go home, except for the newly dead, to attend to the rest of their lives. One more brief paragraph in the history of the troubled country. For the moment, the curiously chaotic events and cataclysmic corrupt revelations of the coming months, involving the precipitate flight of El Chino to Japan and the victory of El Cholo in the subsequent polls, are beyond the capacity of even the most prescient of soothsayers to foretell.

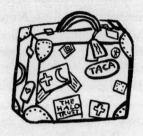

21

Primavera

Springtime. A time for new beginnings. A time of renewal, hope, even miracles. Springtime in Miraflores, the trees in blossom, yellow-flowering *guarango* and orange *tulipana*, the remnants of the Clinic garden at their best, the doves at their busiest and the swooping, squawking parrots at their most scornful. The white-capped nurses are out in the sedate sunshine with their sedentary charges, the D'Onofrio ice cream pedlars emerge with optimism from their winter hibernation, along with Revolución Caliente, the 'hot revolution' ginger biscuit man. Life is full of promise.

'This is Peru,' the Doctor explains. 'Here the people are breathing, living, pumping the pulsating heart.'

May the faltering regime and the devious politicians do their worst, let the greedy bankers reap their just reward. Our business has survived and has new-found financial independence, thanks to the benevolence of the Arequipeño loan. Freed of crippling interest payments, now the Clinic can prosper and the long-awaited lift will be installed; deliveries will take place in the theatre and the upstairs rooms for patients will come to life in a burst of pink and blue ribbon and a profusion of welcoming bouquets. In turn, La Señora's health centres in the suburbs and villages, hitherto but a dream, will develop and flourish to help those in need.

For the Doctor, another season with the bulls at Plaza de Acho is imminent. At El Hipódromo de Monterrico his two new racehorses, Hacker and Espatano, will soon be ready to show their form and, incidentally, the efficacy of Dr Desastre's dynamic equine diets.

Spring fever abounds and at one point I surprise Dr Hermogenes engaged in earnest conversation with a pock-marked, oily-overalled mechanic, both studiously surveying the coachwork of the big, once-white truck. For a fraction of a second I fear that, fired by the all-pervading quickening of the pulses and rising of the sap, a respray is about to return our trusty transport to its pristine glory. The Doctor quickly sets my mind at rest.

'No,' he explains. 'One day we may repaint the wagon and it will look quietly nice. But for the moment, this man he is a technician with knowledge but not too much. He is restricted, he is just the scratch man.'

Well, there are quite a few of those.

For La Señora, it is time again to wield her palette in the atelier at Casa Bonomini; a high-altitude spring exhibition of her paintings is being organized in neighbouring Quito.

'Now I feel so tall and I imagine that, ha! this is my moment! Just think of the advices,' she muses. '"Zapallo-Chupado from Peru presents her paints proudly." I am tired to not sell anything.'

Truly it is a time of awakenings and reawakenings, a time of restlessness.

'I found something back,' declares La Señora. 'In my being, I am a creativity person. Occasionally I put a request on my mind and I thought I was without inspiration because I lost it. I didn't know where was it but now I am painting again. And in these days I paint so good. I can feel the colours in my fingers. When I don't want to, I don't want to, but when I want to, I want to. Sometimes we never know what we have in our reach until we try. When I am in the gallery in Ecuador, you may call me in any moment.'

My work is done, my time has come. In my ears are the siren whispers of the forgotten corners of the world: the high mountains, the empty spaces, the unvisited forests, the distant lands, the false promises of the next valley. After Parcemon's funeral the Doctor had reminded us that we must always be ready with our luggage.

'Be careful of the future,' cautions La Señora. 'We cannot see the future. This suitcase of yours has a lot of stickers. There is no room for more. Stop your luggage here please. Now is not the time to pass into the unknown.' She gazes at the battered case thoughtfully. 'Instead, we need urgently to travel to my stolen land, my hacienda, to see how is the position after a quarter of a century of robbery by presidential decree. In truth I am looking to the future myself now that the Clinic is safe. I want to entrap your imagination, and more, in my next project. I sense the situation in this country is changing and in my mind I am designing a hotel of immense architectural interest and extensive charm within the walls of the great house where once we lived. It will be the quickest of travels,' concludes La Señora, pre-empting the possibility of any objections and casting a gauntlet-glance at the Doctor.

'It will be a "go, see, come trip", yes?' he observes placidly, accepting with outward calm that which he cannot change.

Thus, come what may in the greater scheme of things, it is our moment to visit Puno, albeit fleetingly, before the summer rains fall on the immense tableland of the plateau, 13,000 feet high, those seemingly limitless grasslands of the Altiplano, cradle of the ancient Tiawanaco culture. Modest Puno, on the shores of Lake Titicaca, steeped in history, and the place of La Señora's family hacienda. To fulfil our pilgrimage, we fly to Juliaca, leaving us to travel south by road for less than an hour to reach our destination. In the rickety bus, its chassis distorted and rear axle misaligned so that it proceeds crabwise along the potholed road, we are the only passengers.

'This poor *chofer* that we have,' observes La Señora, 'he tells me that he is a police doing his day off. And just now I think he is hating the people sitting in their warm houses along the way that they are not coming out into the morning to use his bus.'

Next time, we tell ourselves, we may take the train from Arequipa. It is good to believe in next times.

We arrive at the old hacienda, bought, rebuilt and vastly enlarged more than a century ago by La Señora's forebears. The day is crisp and clear, not yet warm, the sharp sunshine falling on the pastureland, countless thousands of hectares where once grazed thousands of sheep, far, far into the distance. And where once, prior to the invidious advent of 'agrarian reform', more than a hundred men had employment, providing their families with food and shelter.

'Now it is all empty,' says La Señora sadly. 'All wasting. But in those days, oh, your eyes couldn't end to see the sheep. Now there is nothing here.'

The mansion, for mansion it is, lies on a small hill, imposing, strongly built in brick to withstand the harsh climate, the heavy roof finished in red tiles. Up the wide steps at the front of the building, we can see into the hall through the open door of the main entrance. At the far end is the grand staircase leading to the living accommodation on the second floor. Amidst the neglect and dust, a few pieces of the original furniture still remain, too heavy to move.

'On that long table there, the men placed their hats when they rode back to the house at the end of the day,' La Señora tells us. 'I remember that we made a new room for the horses; it was not so beautiful but they had no house of their own. Of course, I was not so old, but into this window we can see our dining room. My family we ate and talked there for more than one hundred years. We were a kind family, a worker family. We all helped, I can squeeze a cow. Here it can be very cold at night, always we sat with that big fireplace filled with blazing logs.'

The reminiscences are interrupted by the arrival of an old woman, seemingly drunk, armed with a long-handled scythe to greet us. She speaks only Aymara, the language of the region. But her purpose is clear. It will not be possible to enter La Señora's house today.

'These people are frightened, they know this place it is not theirs. The debt has never been honoured. They came here with envy and because they wanted to say "I climbed up the stairs". Now they do not allow me to get into my house. Perhaps they have no warmth or goodness in their hearts and wish to throw this wonderful house down.'

Led by La Señora we retreat to *la capilla*, the small chapel of the estate, close by on an adjacent fold in the land. Again our way is barred, this time by the padlocked doors. Through the broken windows La Señora can see that the interior has been vandalized.

'I knew this would be so,' she tells us. 'The beautiful Spanish paints and carvings have all been taken.'

There is nothing more for us to see, but before we take our leave of the sadly desolate family hacienda there is a strand of hope. We are joined from nowhere by a nut-brown leather-faced man with twinkling eyes, of uncertain age. His wife brings *maté de coca* from somewhere behind *la capilla* and we sit together by the padlocked doors to catch the sun and share the coca-leaf tea, that altitudinous panacea. Four peach-cheeked children gaze at us in solemn silence as we talk, their bare toes shuffling in the dust.

The man speaks a different message to that of the old woman at the house. 'My name is Baltazar,' he says quietly to La Señora. 'We wish you to come back. We need you here. You must return to your home. Find the way, *por favor*.' His wife and the children look into our eyes. It is springtime, the season of hope and miracles. La Señora believes in next times. And she believes in miracles.

'It is good to dream,' she is in the habit of telling us. 'It makes you grow. From fantasies come beautiful realities. But sometimes your dreams and expectations move too far ahead. So dream on, dream enough but not too much.'

'Yes,' confirms Baltazar, looking into her thoughts. 'In life you will win and you will lose. But always you must hold your head high with dignity. When you know how to live your life, then your life will be beautiful.' And the mystery man with the twinkling eyes gazes peacefully heavenwards at the white clouds and the blue sky above and we learn a new mantra.

'Forget,' he whispers softly. 'Forget the past. The Life goes forward.'

Yes, my work is done. My extended 'six-week' assignment has come to an end. The logic of this escapes La Señora.

'I know how to walk alone but I do not wish to return my jewellery to the crown. I feel that time is pushing us. It is very strange of you. See how important you are that you are making even the maids to cry. Señorita Hilda is distraught, as are the Nurses Dulce and Dolores. As for Ernestina, she has been under the stairs for a week, weeping and inconsolable, smudging the accounts beyond repair. I cannot lie to you about this. You were the image of the Clinic, you were our shining path, our full moon high over the Andes, the sky above our heads. I never brought a British man to be unhappy in my land but why cannot you stay forever? Now you kill me like a fly on top of a *suspiro limeño*, that creamy Lima pudding that is your favourite. Could you please hear to me? Always you have to be cutting your life in the corners. Then, when you turn and look back, there is no one there.'

'Yes. Sometimes it is like that. There is an emptiness. A void.'

'Sometimes? Is that everything once again?'

Maybe La Señora is right, maybe there is no logic. But I am thinking that we need chapters in our lives; chapters that open and close. Either way, she is not pleased and she does not speak for three whole days. In fact, she casually flies off to La Paz for yet another of those wonderful South American weddings.

'I didn't wear too many jewellery,' she relates on her return. 'And how long ago I don't see you. Everyone was in short dresses just to pass the night but I was in long, in the very latest mood. I was the show of the evening. I enter to these long stairs and the Doctor he was very proud of me. The bride's mother, she is in the jail at present. It is political and financial, but she comes out often and was at home for the wedding. And now let me explain you this. There is one thing more you need to understand and that is when here we say that I am not going to talk to you any more again, twenty minutes later we are talking. It is because we are Latins.'

Serendipitously, during her travels the altitude has prompted La Señora's mind to perceive a not-to-be-missed opportunity to stage on my behalf *una fiesta de despedida*, a farewell extravaganza of immense proportions and incomparable jollity. Indeed, an occasion of such overwhelming happiness that she will undoubtedly enjoy the luxury of shedding *coco-drilo* tears throughout the proceedings at the unbearable and exquisite sadness of it all.

'It's good that we resolved our differences,' I remark, taking advantage of La Señora's change in spirits.

'No,' she rebukes. 'Better if they had never occurred. But don't talk back about that. The noble people is not reminding the bad things. I notice that a little bit in you. Now we must use this moment that we are in.'

'Who shall be invited?'

After seventy-two hours of silence I am momentarily surprised by La Señora's question.

'Hilmutt Cup-Head, the one-eared barman,' I reply.

'And Abraham the scissor-dancing butler and Margarita the laughing black cook,' adds La Señora. 'They are for the drinking and the eating. Now for the talking and the dancing?'

'Chichi Peralta and Willy Colón,' I say, naming two of my favourites. 'That's for the dancing. For the talking, perhaps the same as the Christmas party?'

'But without the Russians and the Swedes and obviously without Papá Noel. They are not springtime persons.'

'So that will leave room for Fabiolita, Lillianita, Charapita, Teresita, Tortalita, Carmencita, Cecilita, Romanita, Ingridsita, Sashacita and Picaflor, the well-fitted ladies in the leotards from *el gimnasio*? And even Flor de Loto.' Then I suggest somewhat tentatively, 'And possibly the Hungry Poetess, as an act of kindness to ease her loneliness?'

'*¿Qué?* Who?'

'Er, and Big Pepe from *el gimnasio* who can lift two hundred kilograms with one hand and also Inti Raymi Pepe who went to Cusco and paradoxically and perversely spent a whole week celebrating the Day of the Sun, that renowned Inca festival. And his friendly friend, Raphael.'

'If that's what you want. Altogether we shall have a beautiful participation in the party. And all the family of course.'

The Committee, of course, so that we may anticipate another excellent crop of character assassinations, the demolition of yet more reputations.

'And Simon,' I add.

'Simon?' La Señora frowns. 'Is he strong too? Simons are not normally so strong. Or is he just perverse?'

'No, he's not from the gym. He's from my other church, the Cathedral of the Good Shepherd. He supports Manchester City.'

'Is that good? Is he a saint?'

'Very nearly, it's just a question of time. The point is, there aren't many of us, and even fewer in Peru.'

'As you wish,' says La Señora. 'If it's an environmental thing, invite him. I do not understand everything in this life.'

No need to invite the Yorkies. They will come anyway and pee against the table legs and into the shoes of the guests. And even cock an affectionate leg over long-suffering Carlos, the tormented transsexual tortoise, formerly Carlotta.

Ordering a meal in a restaurant and organizing a party on the grandest of scales: these are two things that La Señora can do without moving her lips. It is magical to behold. In the latter case, up goes *el toldo*, the bedecked durbar marquee, out go the gregariously rounded tables, each with its attendant shapely cluster of curved-back chairs, in come the music men with big black speakers, microphones and miles of cables. What else? All the impedimenta necessary for a sumptuous feast are laid in place, a profusion of expensively exuberant flowers is pleasingly arranged, golden lamps are lit. And not a word is spoken. La Señora ignores the whole unseemly process as unworthy of her attention, at a time when most hostesses might be inclined to fuss and fret and even to get ever-so-slightly involved in the preparations. No, for La Señora it is sufficient to sweep down the stairs of Casa Bonomini in tiara, crown jewels and the most graceful of gowns two hours after the appointed time. And that she does supremely well.

Doing equally well is Dr Hermogenes, dispensing his pisco sours. Aunt Gertrudis is also looking well, as do most people when bearing two brimming bottles of bubbling best *brut* champagne. Yes, all the ingredients for yet another successful party are in place and successful it is. Dr Desastre, dearly beloved, is one of the last guests to arrive; rubicund Rudecindo is one of the first.

'Are you really departing?' asks rubicund Rudecindo absently. 'If so,' he continues, 'this I may not have told you before,' throwing back his third pisco sour so fast that, like the first and second, it doesn't touch the sides, 'but before the disaster of agrarian reform my family had lands that reached from *la costa* through *la sierra* to *la selva*.'

'Goodness me!' I exclaim. 'From the coast across the mountains to the jungle! You must have needed a private railway to travel from one side to the other.'

'How did you know that?' enquires rubicund Rudecindo suspiciously, troubling Hilmutt Cup-Head for yet another pisco but overlooking the fact that Hilmutt's only ear is on the other side of his head, with the result that Hilmutt goes untroubled and thirsty Rudecindo goes untended.

As guest of honour I have had my hour, I am yesterday's man. Like the bride and groom at the wedding feast, my presence has become incidental. 'Thank you for providing the excuse for this splendid occasion,' say the guests, 'but *con permiso*, excuse us, now we need to get on with the fun. By the way, have a good journey to wherever it is, and do drop by again soon. And is that Willy Colón we hear playing?' Ta-ta-ta taa-taa. Da-da-da daa-daa! 'Everybody on the dance floor!' And dance we do, until goodness knows when, never mind the neighbours. I know that the time is goodness-knows-when never-mind-the-neighbours because rubicund Rudecindo reappears at my elbow. He eyes my favourite tie ominously, the one with the large pink spots that my Aunt Agripina, may she rest in peace, gave me for my birthday long ago when the world was young.

'This I may not have told you before,' he says predictably, in a sibilance of spray, the words slithering out of the side of his mouth in that special late-night style of his, 'but your tie is like chicken's balls.'

'That is a biological improbability,' I reply, with just a hint of the old English toffee in my voice.

'Sorry, I mean chicken pox,' explains rubicund Rudecindo hurriedly, unusually chastened. And off he sways to make new friends.

At lunchtime the following day I am preparing to leave the Clinic for the very last time, on my way to find some breakfast in Casa Bonomini, when by chance Medical Student Two appears.

'Hmmmm,' he says equivocally. 'I see you not too well today.'

And with this supportive pronouncement, he is gone again, off on his nefarious errands.

Undeterred, I leave my bulging suitcase, roped and ready to journey into the unknown, on the balcony overlooking the auditorium outside my diminutive roof-top room and, accompanied by the splash and tinkle of the water-feature waterfall, embark on a final tour of my parish.

It occurs to me that the new lift will give Aunt Gertrudis renewed after-lunch access to the fourth floor, thus facilitating her reinstatement as Executive Controller, so I visit my office to ensure that all is in order for her comfortable occupancy. I wonder if before I leave I ought to install a cocktail cabinet for her as a farewell present. Thus engaged, I am startled by the soft footfall of Señorita Hilda.

'I will miss you,' she declares, unexpectedly. We look at each other in surprise and then, together, we look out through the window and study the dead tree, symbol of we are not sure what. For once, the pigeons are still and silent and, heads enquiringly askew, they blink, or wink, at us in encouragement.

'What happened to the new intercom system?' I ask, clumsily, to fill the gap.

Señorita Hilda turns the page, perhaps closing the chapter, and takes the enquiry in her stride. 'The headphones and aerials are in the store-room for whenever we need them. But for the moment, La Señora has decided that it will be easier if we talk to each other without them, you know, normally.' Then she shifts the heavy weight of her peripatetic paperwork from under one arm to the other. 'Anyway, *con permiso*, I must be getting along.' And like Medical Student Two, she also disappears from my life.

In the aptly named Patient Reception, Dr Ching is on the point of departure, hurrying off to his laboratory to analyse the contents of his sandwich box. He gives a Chinese chuckle, shakes me enthusiastically by the hand, head nodding the whilst, and he too is gone. It is one of those days. Nurses Dulce and Dolores gaze at me with glistening eyes. I try not to glisten back.

'I will look after your garden for you,' promises Nurse Dulce. 'Before, when we lived in the mountains, I helped my father.'

I nod in appreciation of the longest speech that Nurse Dulce has ever made, grateful that perhaps, for once, this is a garden that will not die with the gardener. Even though, with La Señora's help, it nearly died in advance of my passing.

'And I can wind your cuckoo clock,' offers Nurse Dolores, hopefully, also in loquacious mood. 'Every morning I have watched you do it.'

Again I nod vigorously. The more these two talk, the fewer words I have. And again, I am grateful. It is good to know that time will not stop when I leave.

Under the stairs, Ernestina is expecting me, busily applying finishing touches to her new account book, wrist looped in that curious curve favoured by the left-handed in an endeavour to see what they are writing, pending the day when as one they rise in revolt and thenceforth start to scribe from right to left.

'Look,' she says proudly, revealing the almost immaculate ledger. 'I have prepared it exactly like you showed me. Everything entered into the correct columns. Hardly any crossings-out and no crumbs at all. Now, whenever you return, this will be ready and you can teach me how to put everything on to the computer, just as you said. Then we can throw these big books in the cupboard. Yes?' She looks up at me through her wide, trusting spectacles, so that I am impelled to take refuge in the Victorian tea-room.

'You are leaving?' enquires Dr Vonday, putting down his truffle with careful precision to preclude as far as practicable the unwanted dislodgement of any of the adhering chocolate particles and at the same time coming perilously close to verging on a state of mild interest and animation.

'Yes. But I'll be back. One day.' I add the last bit to save him the trouble.

'*Ja*,' he says, disappointingly. 'Dr Cleeber is operating at the moment but I will tell him you passed by.'

La Señora and Dr Hermogenes take me to catch my flight. The luggage of my life is ready: the battered suitcase, magic carpet of my travels, veteran of one hundred and one adventures into the unknown. Held together by rope and the legacy of colourful labels, it lies unemotionally in the back of the big, once-white, now scratch-free truck. The case is full, jammed with the material clutter of my Peruvian idyll, the criffle-cruffle of mementos. I sit on the long front seat between the Doctor and La Señora. My mind is also full, packed with a thousand thoughts, a thousand memories. This is where it all started. Can this really be our last journey to Jorge Chávez Airport? Always believe in next time.

Peruvians never say 'goodbye'. It is not the way, the implied finality is not to be countenanced. *Adiós* is not goodbye, it is God's blessing. God be with you. *Gracias a Dios*, thanks to God. 'Until the next time, until later, until then,' that's what they say. *Hasta la próxima, hasta luego, hasta la vista*. The door is ajar, the candle burning bright, the kettle simmering on the hearth for your return, your *maté de coca* ready on the table. 'Please pour my tea,' they say, 'and keep my cup to await my return.' Next time. One day.

'Enjoy your holiday,' says La Señora Coraima Pandora del Teodosia Zapallo-Chupado Palermo Bonomini. 'The cuckoo clock will beat the moments until you return and I will call you when I am ready.'

'Holiday? Ready?' Not those midnight calls again.

'*Sí*, when I am ready then I will call. Surely you remember that we have been invited back to my hacienda in Puno? It is our next endeavour.'

Dr Hermogenes Abelardo Abasalon shrugs and rolls his eyes. Then he gathers strength. With all those undulating hectares there has to be room somewhere for a few bulls and horses. Happily, it will be too high for ostriches. Surely?

La Señora repeats herself above the silence. 'I will call you when I am ready.'

'Yes,' I hear myself reply. 'Yes, call me and I will come. Wait for me.'

'Is that a Peruvian "yes" or a British "yes"?'

'Just blow a kiss across the ocean and I will come.'

'*Gracias*. Thank you to you.' La Señora holds me in her eyes. 'Come as soon as you can, if not before.' Then she turns to the Doctor and to no one in particular. 'We lost him,' she whispers. 'I never knew he would leave the tea so fast, the cup he left upon the table is getting cold and now the wind is blowing through the open door. When the candle flickers, so the friendship flickers and if the flame dies then I will know that he has gone from here for ever. He will be lost to us on the winds and tides of eternity and he will go we know not where.'

It is a moment for keeping stiff the upper lip. A farewell is like a rehearsal for a funeral.

'Whatever happens,' I proclaim boldly, paraphrasing that fearless young aviator, the tragically romantic Jorge Chávez, 'I shall be found on the other side of the Andes.' And with a nonchalant wave of the hand to belie the forlorn heaviness of my heart and the depth of sadness in my soul, I am gone. A feather in the wind.

Acknowledgements

With especial gratitude to Hazel Wood for her wise, untiringly diplomatic and inspirational support; to Caroline Knox for her judgement and faith; to Oliver Lane for his invaluable professional contribution and suggestions; to Caroline Westmore for her advice and help on manifold aspects and occasions; to Dominic Lane for his unfailing in-depth response to research requests, invariably at short notice; and to Elizabeth Dobson, copy editor and master of her craft.

In conclusion, with much appreciation to British Executive Service Overseas, under whose auspices the author originally went to Lima (and indeed, to many other parts of the world).